HIV/AIDS
Why Me?

Is ah chance ah go take

Karcian Suragh

This book is a work of fiction based on real events that occurred over a period of time. Any resemblance to persons, living or dead, or places, events or locales is purely coincidental. The characters were real at some point in time but are still a re-production of the author's imagination.

Adult Reading Material

ISBN Number: 9798842208258

Acknowledgements

To my sons
    Jobari Suragh
    Jadon Suragh

My nephew
    Jovan Thomas

Table of Contents

Foreword

"When I first met the author Mr. Karcian Suragh I was present-
ed with one hundred plus pages to type, which was the work of
this heart. My objective, to take his raw draft and create a word
document, format for a printer and complete all illustrations. I
accepted the challenge gladly, little did I know that in these pages
would contain not only a story but the untold voices and souls of
the HIV epidemic. This disease is still taboo among many of us.
It's never really foremost on our minds because we convince ourselves that we aren't the type of person who gets AIDS, because we
aren't doing anything wrong. Surely, those who have it did something to deserve it. We even believe it is still a homosexual disease,
nevertheless Karcian has been able to prove most unequivocally
in this compilation that the disease is opportunistic and without
prejudice to every sexual orientation. It occurred to me while
completing this project that one of the most hidden symptoms of
the HIV virus is an increase in the desire for sex - so the act that
creates it, fuels it and then becomes it's demise. This book is about
you and I, our family and friends, our neighbours and co-workers;
normal, average people that we meet everyday. Every time I completed a story I envision that this soul who roamed the pages was
now at rest. I understand now why the author feels intensely about
printing this book because at long last, he is honouring them,
honouring their journey. This book should not be considered as
an expose of sorts or an invasion of privacy nor a tool of gossip,
but a more so, what it is, a tribute to those whose lives were stuffed
out prematurely. This book is a must read for every man, woman
and teen, anyone who is having sex or thinking about having sex.
There is no real guide to safe sex but this book provides a much
needed awareness and perspective as we continue to wage and win
the battle against the disease."

Marsha Gomes-Mckie, Founder, Caribbean Books Foundation

The decision with the moment of pleasure can be a lifetime of pain.

Introduction

What is HIV?
The human immunodeficiency virus (HIV) is a virus that attacks the immune system, the body's natural defence system, without a strong immune system the body has trouble fighting off diseases, both the virus and the infection it causes are called HIV.
www.vaccines.gov

What is AIDS?
1. AIDS stands for Acquired Immune Deficiency Syndrome
2. Acquired means you can get infected with it.
3. Immune Deficiency means a weakness in the body's system that try to fight off diseases that can make other conditions develop such as cancer and allows pneumonia to thrive.
4. Syndrome means a group of multiple health problems that help make up the disease.
www.aidsinfo.org

"My name is Karcian Ekron Suragh, for starters I am not an author of many books nor do I have much experience at all in writing books. People, while reading I hope and pray that you may learn a lesson from these stories. There are not many words to replace or substitute more than the original ones, fiction I can add but true and real stories such as these must be told as is.

What has been written from start to finish is not fictionalized nor is it of any imagination from my mind. These events speak of actual places with real people who are either living or dead. As a matter of fact, this book clearly shows a wide range of risk and behaviour of persons who took great chances with their lives. Each and every person in these stories was a very close and dear friend of mine.

Thereafter, you will be able to see that in situations like these no one is perfect or has a shield of covering around them. No one is invincible, it matters not whether you are black, white, Spanish, Indian, Chinese; man or woman; boy or girl; rich or poor, this can happen to any one of us as human beings.

Everything that has been imparted, with the best of my knowledge is what actually happened. For reasons of privacy the characters and places have been renamed, to protect the individuals who are still alive. In other stories a skit has been used to get my point across where trini[1] men and women cheat on each other, in our own words, it is a language of 'horning'[2]. Each and every event took place some odd fifteen years or more ago. This book was written using dialect or plain trini slang. Some of the words were the actual words used by persons and was documented how it was spoken.

On HIV/AIDS risk and behaviour of the human kind, my knowledge is limited in that area so I can only explain briefly the personal impact. I hope the characters and sound of the words used may be understandable for the learning purpose of cultural reason and indifference. My closing statement is that the decision in the moment of pleasure can be a lifetime of pain.

1 A person born in Trinidad and Tobago
2 To be unfaithful in your relationship

Our culture in Trinidad and Tobago is cosmopolitan, people of mixed race from every background of nations worldwide. The percentage of ethnic groups seems to be changing rapidly, the exact amount may be untold. These are just some of the estimated numbers below:

40%	African descent (Black/Creole)
42%	East Indian descent (Indian)
16%	Mixed Race
0.8%	Caucasian descent (White)
1.2%	Asian and Other descent(Chinese)

"When Indian meets Creole we does make Dougla children, Black and White we making Mulatto children, Mixed Spanish, Amerindian, Afro-Latino is Coco-payols. You getting White and Black Mulatto giving you French Creole Children, is Chinese and White Caucasian, Portuguese and Syrian, Black Carib and White Mixed Brown skin, Latino mixed, the list goes on and on and if you ask me what the rest of them is called I don't have a clue. To begin we are a callalloo kind of people and hot blooded so if the excitement of sex comes upon us where we have to make a choice between a plate of food and a naked woman, I strongly believe the plate of food will take second place."

Apart from all of this we are a very happy people in the blue Caribbean Sea and all are continued to be welcomed."

Mr. Fabulous

"This is the beginning of a journey past and present where I have seen people from all creed and race including good friends and relatives living and dead with HIV/AIDS. This deadly beast of disease can come with a single man or woman which may circulate into groups beyond and countless numbers of any amount. What does this mean? The story you are about to read is not glamorous in any form or fashion of any kind, it was not handed down information, I was present with each and every individual at the time. I hope that you gain some knowledge and understanding while reading.

It all started with just one man, Mr. Fabulous. He was a very clever, conniving, and intelligent person who was well known to me and many others. If you see him during those times gone by, he did not look as an HIV infected person.

Mr. Fabulous used to be well dressed. He was short and stocky built, dark complexion, not too good looking in his white vest and three quarter pants, with his Marvin Gaye hat on his head together with matching colours of socks and clean shoes. He was always smelling sweet but couldn't hide the bad breath, he forever had a broad smile that showed his white teeth. Like any one else he was very friendly, yet he tend to talk a lot with his body, touching his gold chain, adjusting the gold on his fingers and hands so you could pay attention to it.

Every morning before work he would go outside of the building to position himself on the road-way watching every lady that passed by, most of them would stop and chat with him on their way to work. Now this was a good way to lure them into him, not all women are the same but most of the girls now would love a bling man[3], a bad man of sorts, a gangsta man, a rude boy as they say. He used to say quite regularly, "Ha ha ha it must be that yuh done know ha ha ha." I never really knew what was the meaning of that slang but the girls loved it and was all over him. I watched his every move and every one that was involved with him on the same compound. Most of the girls never used condoms, some of these girls at the time were young girls going to school while others were working married women or common law[4] women in steady relationships who were already living with a man.

Please stay with me here, every one of these women would give him a phone number to make contact with them at the end of the day, during the day or on weekends. Mr. Fabulous was a good tracker[5] man as they say, with words to seduce and funniness to make you laugh out loud. He was full of jokes and soon he captured his prey, once he got you into that spot, that kind of mood, I believed that you were as good as dead.

Within that same compound where we were, I also saw many women and girls got caught up in that sex circle. There were two sisters that Mr. Fabulous was with at the same time. The older

---

3 A person who wears large gold items for show
4 Someone you live with, you are not married to but in Trinidad due to the number of years together they can have a legal claim as a spouse
5 Someone who seduces ladies easily

sister would go to his home and they would cook together early on, then she'd take the food to work and set up to sell in her shop. Now the man also had a sweet hand even I ate from him, he was a good cook. While the older sister was in her shop he would leave and go meet the younger sister in a hotel of choice to have sex without the other one knowing. It was very interesting how he did this because those two girls had their own shop and would take turns holding on for each other in the shop not knowing that both of them was dealing with the same man. This situation went on for years and years, I really don't know how it carried on so long but as I remember I will write.

While dealing with the both of them at the same time without either one knowing Mr. Fabulous started feeling sick and was in and out of the hospital but no one knew why or what was wrong with him. This went on for two weeks straight, I asked him what was wrong with him and he noted that it was shingles because there was a rash on his face. I didn't think it was a problem.

These girls, the two sisters started worrying, when they asked him what the problem was, why he was in and out of the hospital he told them that it was a routine check-up; that the doctors said to check into the hospital every now and again and it wasn't serious. The following week he got ill again and was hospitalized for another two weeks, but this time he discharged himself and came home. Upon arrival he looked different, his Marvin Gaye hat was low on his head and his socks was all the way up his feet to his pants. When I made investigations as to the reason he was dressing like that I was told it was to cover up some sores that was coming out on his body. He also went to the toilet and wash room many times for the day, this went on for a while. Then he seemed to get everything under control.

Stay with me, I will come back to tell you the rest of the story with the two sisters but first let me follow the story as it goes and introduce myself to you.

One morning, I went to the shop and Ms. Helen told me that she' was in love with me and it was right time for me to know her feelings towards me, since she'd been keeping it in a long time. While we spoke Helen asked me to come downstairs and open the gate for her to get inside the shop the next morning at 6 am.

I agreed, it wasn't a problem to help Helen so the next morning I woke early as promised and went to open the gate. It was my intention to go back upstairs after doing so but she asked me to stay in the shop with her with a big smile.

"Why, for what? " I asked.

"To keep me company," Helen grinned.

"Okay but only for a minute," I agreed.

We both sat on a long puffy looking couch thing and talked, I can say temptation is a hell of a thing, if you cannot control yourself.

It was not a good two minutes before Helen asked me, "Do you want to see something?"

"See what?"' I asked like a fool.

Then she asked me again. I said yes of course show me something. The woman put one leg up in a seated position while the other one was down and she began spreading her legs apart asking me if ah seeing it and to come closer and look.

"Take it now," she teased. "Take it when you could get it now is the chance."

Now I wasn't seeing anything from my view but the woman had on no underwear, unknown to me, my children's mother was peeping through a hole in the flooring at us.

"Look someone peeping at us," Helen hissed.

"Whey," I asked.

"Look up," Helen replied.

I looked up only to see an eye looking straight at us, then the eye disappeared. Seconds after my children's mother was standing in Helen's doorway glaring like a mad bull.

Oh boy, look trouble, look bacchanal. "Ah catch yuh, boy yuh mother so and so, I go fxxk you up, what you doing here early in the morning by this bitch shop eh? Then, "girl I best beat yuh ass for you?"
Helen tried to plead, "but we was not doing anything."

"You was not doing anything, opening up your legs for my man, telling him to see and come closer, yuh bitch, yuh blasted whore like you.

Okay to avoid any further problems I went back upstairs with my children's mother where I belonged.

The next day Helen and I took a chance to speak about she wanting to give me some loving out of the blue, just so, knowing that I was living upstairs with my children and their mother. I explained to her that once I was living with someone I didn't fool around and I was not the kind of man to do such things. She said it was okay.

Somehow something was not right with Helen, she too changed. To my knowledge she would lock up shop and leave every day at 3 o'clock on evenings, I watched her movements good one day only to observe Mr. Fabulous, on the same compound lock up and leave right after Helen. It became a pattern. Just a little way from the building, a block away I saw both Miss Helen and Mr. Fabulous holding hands, walking together down the street as real lovers do.

Apart from Helen and before previous situations Mr. Fabulous had two children mothers. One of them totally cut him off by stopping the relationship but the other one was still sleeping with him. There were times when she needed money for her son, she would come and start quarrelling and fighting, mashing up almost everything in his shop until I got involved by being in the middle of both parties having to make arrangements with him to collect the money and take it out the building for her to collect, in order to prevent confusion between them.

Take note how many women he was involved with at the same time and the list goes on and on.

I then saw Mr. Fabulous going out with Helen. Miss Helen who professed how much she adored me, which for me was not of interest. She and Mr. Fabulous were in a sexual fling or relationship of sorts, apart from that I noticed my neighbour Keith sweet on Helen. They were caught going to a hotel to have sex. This was at the same time that she was in the sexual relationship with Mr. Fabulous, both men knew one another and she would have had me to if I wanted to get involved and so the sex circle continues.

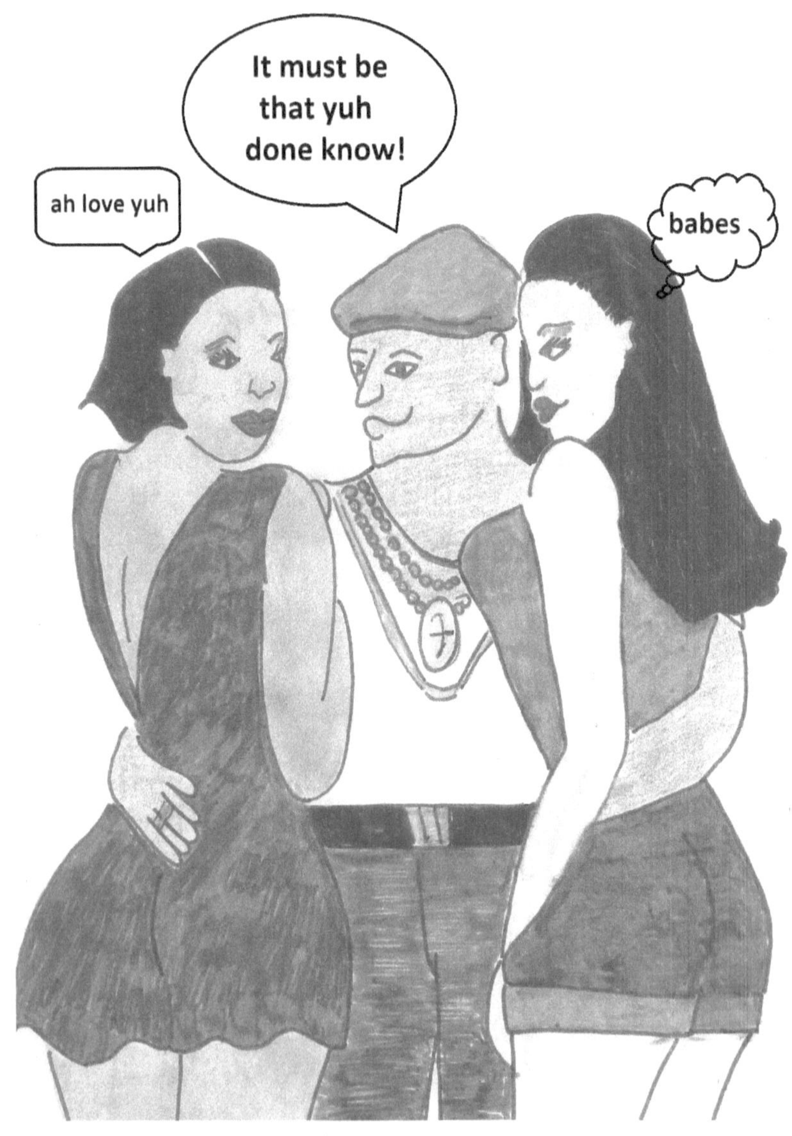

It must be
that yuh
done know!
ah love yuh
babes

Keith my neighbour upon reaching home would have a girl waiting in his bed to have sex. She would leave very early before daylight and return to her apartment, since she was also a neighbour. Kate, lived just above me and according to the night she would go across to Keith multiple times to have sex.

There was another friend of my sister to whom I am very familiar with, her name is Brenda. Both my sister and I knew Brenda for many years and to our surprise she was seen going home by Keith occasionally. We meet a few times and spoke.

"This is not my business to judge you," I would say. "But what are you doing home by Keith?"

She smiled, which was her usual thing and admitted that they were dealing[6] for about two years or more.

Watch the picture here: Mr. Fabulous is having sex with one of his children's mother, one of them cut the relationship the other one stays. He is also sleeping with two sisters, without either one knowing then he is having sex with Helen, who is sleeping with Keith too. Kate is home waiting for Keith every night to have sex and Brenda is going to Keith's to have sex at a different time. Brenda was in a relationship with Keith for two years or more having sex without either of them knowing. All these girls were being played in a circle of fake relationships.

Nevertheless Kate broke off the sexual relationship she was having with Keith and found real love, with someone else, she is married with children now. Mr. Fabulous children mother, the one who mashed up his shop, found out about the entire situation and the relationship came to an end.

<u>Don't stop read</u>ing. Still in the building is another woman who

6 *In a sexual relationship*

is married and one of the sisters, the younger one is going out with her husband, taking him to hotels to have sex with him while his wife await his return. The younger sister would drop him lower down the road where he would walk back to his wife normal, normal as nobody business. This married man would tell his wife, "Honey ah going down the road and come back."

She would answer, "Okay love, be safe."

This went on for a good while, at the same time I saw my best friend's wife hanging out at Mr. Fabulous. I may lose count with the women here. When I ask her what are you doing over there by Mr. Fabulous? She turned and smiled, which anyone could see and know already what was going on with her. Then one day, she ask me for my phone number.

"Why do you want my number?" I asked.

She said with a smile, "you will see."

A couple of days after she did call, told me I'm being invited home for dinner. Why and what happened to your husband who is my best friend, I inquired. She said calmly that they were separated for some time now. Hold on, this is how the story went and there is no other way it can be told.

My best friend name was 'Bagoboy, we were friends for years and he also knew of Mr. Fabulous. They were very good buddies but I could of never tell or say for sure if he was dealing with one of the two sisters. Here it was on Monday morning very early about 7:30 a.m. that he came to me in desperation and anxiety hoping that the answer to the question was no. So 'Bagoboy told me upfront that he love this girl so much, they've been together for a while and he made proposal marry her.

"The reason why I love this girl," this man told me over and over how much he cared for her. How she'd sleep by his house every weekend and clean, wash and cook for him but on Monday she would leave.

So 'Bagoboy became curious and followed her that Monday morning after she spent the weekend by him. He could not believe his eyes when she entered the compound.

The question he asked me of course was that if every Monday morning his girl friend, after she left by him would come down there, to this building.

"Yes," I answered, "but how would I know you were involved with this girl. I am now getting to know about this one."

He asked me once again if when she leave by him on Monday morning if she does come here every time.

"Do you want to know the answer?" I asked him.

"Yes," he proclaimed.

But each time I begin to tell him, what I wanted to tell him he would say. "Doh tell meh nah." When I made another attempt he just kept on saying, "doh tell meh, please doh tell meh."

Eventually, after an hour I said to him, we can't keep up this childish behaviour. When he calmed down a bit, and started listening to what I had to say, I was able to say. "You are my good friend right."

He nodded and said yes.

"You want to know," I continued. "If this girl you sleeping with is with your good friend Mr. Fabulous right?"

It was not nice when he got the news that every Monday morning when he was finished with her, that this is where she came and met Mr. Fabulous. After hearing the news I could not keep him quiet, at that point he started banging his head on the walls, then he put his both hands on his head, walked a good way up from the building sat in the hot sun and cried out continuously. "Oh God, Oh God, Oh God, Oh my Lord, Lord, Lord!"

What a surprise to me now since this was the younger sister, the one out of the two sisters who was going out with the married man, she played both men, he and my best friend and she was still with the man himself, Mr. Fabulous.

Next in this vicious circle is my padner's[7] brother whose name was Carter. I had known both men for some years, well Carter was a trades man doing construction for a living, if things got slow at times he would ply[8] his car on the road for hire. Now Carter was a popular man for having many different lady friends, not that he was a player but if things didn't work out where the relationship was concerned between both parties, he would make changes very quickly. Carter was a cool and pleasant person, one day he brought a very nice young lady and introduced her to me saying: "This is the one."

"Are you sure?" I asked him.

"Yes," he said. "She is the last one, after her there is no one else. This is the real one because I am going to marry her."

---

7 *Male friend*
8 *To use a private car as a taxi for hire*

"Once you are sure," I said, "that's great."
So Carter and his wife to be started making wedding arrangements for the near future. A couple of months down the road they give me a wedding invitation, which I gladly accepted. This wedding was to take place the next year but I was prepared to go because I was happy for this man, I thought it was time for him to settle down and stop changing women like underwear. Things were good for them, Carter was happy with his new girlfriend and all was well. One day Carter's brother paid me a visit only to say Carter girlfriend fall real sick and ended up in the hospital and when the doctors do a test she was diagnosed with the HIV virus and AIDS; she was already so gone, but she never took a test because she did not know at the time what was going on. His wife to be passed away. I cannot say how long she lasted but the doctors made a phone call to Carter asking him to come for an HIV test. He did visit the hospital, he took the test and doctors confirmed that Carter had contracted the HIV virus from his wife to be. He stood watching in a daze he couldn't believe what he was hearing. Apparently after a moment his brother said to him; "Please let me take you by a lady, she may be able to help you."

He didn't hear anything his brother was saying to him, this man walk all the way from the hospital to home in disbelief and shock. He locked himself up in the house not wanting to see anyone, no one, not even me, he wasn't eating or drinking water, nothing at all. Eventually he died, one year later from starvation and dehydration. Knowing what had happened to him, all the stress, I just did not think he could have lived with himself anymore so he gave up on life.

Now watch the picture here, Carter who wanted to marry his new girlfriend, the girl who he had shown to me, the one who he introduced as his wife to be with the invitation and wedding arrangements, with all that excitement, this same girl was with Mr. Fabulous long before Carter meet her. It was as Mr. Fabulous said: Ha ha ha, it must be that you done know.

As I continue into another story it's like a chain reaction of events. We move on to a man by the name, Mazda man. Mazda man was the main taxi driver on the road, he was a favourite, a very special one among the school girls because he played loud, hard-pound[9] music in his car. Very soon he was nicknamed Soundman. So Soundman would pick up school girls back and forth from school each and every day as he ply-ed his taxi, which most of the time would be half-working, half falling apart and broken down especially when you are near your destination.

Yes he was a friendly guy with manners and courtesy to every one that was in contact with him. Soundman would change cars very often due to the nature of problems, that he may have with one or another vehicle for example his vehicles smoked a lot from the exhaust when driving but somehow the girls were attracted to this man and his troublesome cars. They would wait on him every day, I don't know the reason why or could not understand why, but whatever he was doing worked fine for them. If I told you the truth, Soundman would never dress good, most of the time he would be shaggy looking, dirty looking and smelling rusty. Some people sat next to him just to go home and dealt with it because you have to bear with it to reach home, don't talk about when the rain fall and he wound up his glass with no air-conditioning, is now people would dead in that car.

One day while travelling with Soundman he said to me; "Boy, I don't know but ah feeling that ah was with one of them girls who was dealing with Mr. Fabulous."

---

9 *Extremely loud music*

"Are you telling me or asking me?" I replied but he didn't respond.

It was a little while down the road, a period of some months where I had not seen Soundman or heard of him. Someone who knew him told me that he had a bad stroke from taking a bath with cold water from a barrel that was covered down behind his house.

Knowing me of course, I went to look for him, after meeting we chatted about his condition and what happened. He then repeated what he told me before that he thought he had sex with one of the girls who was with Mr. Fabulous.

"Did you use a condom?" I asked.

"No," he said. "I can't remember."

"Did you go get tested for HIV?' I continued.

"No," he responded again.

"So how will you know for sure if you have contracted the disease?" I probed.

"I am not going to be tested or to take treatment, okay," he replied.

"The ball is in your court, do what you feel is right," I said as I left.

I cannot judge a man but he became more ill and was in a rotten, smelly situation until no other driver wanted Soundman to travel with him in their car. So he would walk up and walk back down again in whatever way that he could when he had to go somewhere.

"Why aren't you going for medication?" I would ask whenever I saw him.

"Ah-go-go, when ah ready," was his response.

Some people you really have to leave them alone. However it took him some time but he eventually went to take the test, his results was positive and yes, when he found out he knew it was one of the school girls. Soundman's friend, Mr. Fabulous was with all of the school girls before him. He told me the real problem was he could not remember which one of the school girls gave him the HIV virus because he had sex with too many of them without a condom. Since then I have not seen nor heard from Soundman, I don't know if he is dead or alive.

I am going to conclude this story of Mr. Fabulous in a while but I must continue with the two sisters and how both of them were with him without the other one knowing.

After spending the two weeks in the hospital where he discharged himself it was not long again that he was warded, this trip he was too weak to stand or work so the doctors recommended bed rest with drips, he was to remain hospitalized.

Upon reaching the hospital at whatever ward he was in during visiting hours, one of the sisters moved hastily towards the bedside of Mr. Fabulous, wanting to know anxiously what was wrong with him. When she saw the doctors they pulled her to one side and said to her: "You have to know what is going on with your man, the reason why he is in and out of the hospital regularly, your man Mr. Fabulous is dying with AIDS."

Just how she get the news quickly, she ran out from the hospital and was on her way back to the building where we were. I was right next door as she approached her sister, I could have seen the expression on their faces.

"Girl you know what that man have?" She croaked.

"Please tell meh, tell meh nah, tell me girl," she asked again. "De man dying with what?"

"The doctor say AIDS, AIDS!" Her sister shouted.

Then the house came down.

"Oh no, oh no, oh no, oh my God," She cried out loud.

What a nightmare, those screams were heard throughout the entire building and people came running to the rescue as if it was a robbery taking place.

Then people were asking what happened to you?

"Nothing, nothing,"

"Really you sure?"

"Yeah ah good," she said to them while I stood my ground and watched the horror unfold. Up to this day these two sisters are unsettled, knowing what had taken place.

The older of the two was living with her personal boyfriend and was still involved in a relationship with Mr. Fabulous, at the same time, for a few years well. After her boyfriend heard about <u>Mr. Fabulous </u>and how his girlfriend was dealing[10] with him the

10 *Having Sex*

man wasted no time, he took rope, tied it to the roof of their house and jumped to his death. The younger sister airbrushed a tattoo on the ankle of her foot, it's a vine which is visible to the eye that runs right up under her skirt, if you need to see the flowers you will have to go to bed with her to see the promise land of no return, which most men would do almost anything to go there.

This is the final on Mr. Fabulous life expectancy, due to his condition he has now become worse, on his way out, bedridden, the doctors pleaded and begged of him to give us the names of all the girls he had sex with. He was a bit hesitant to speak but he eventually did, after the doctors received the names they made phone calls. They called each one of the girls telling them to come for an HIV test while receiving the message their mother's cried out loud together with their daughters. My next door neighbour was one of them this was not easy to hear much less to deal with, but it happened.

This is how the story went and no other way in which it could be told, he had been dealing with each and every girl and woman at the same time. Just different days in the month of the year. How he did it no one could tell, only him alone knew, not even his child mother the one that used to fight with him and break up all his stuff had a clue. As they say behind closed doors no one sees but God apparently. They were still together for a while, with him knowing what was going on with his health but she never knew of his condition at any given time. Within a period between the relationship she became sick and was hospitalized and remained there and died. They had a son long before he contracted the HIV virus. His good friend who shared sex with the younger sister 'Bagoboy had no time to take a test and medication, he died in a car accident by a broken neck.

There was a Minister at the bedside of Mr. Fabulous speaking to him while he lay helpless in his bed with drips running down his already shrunken body, his nose on his face was no more, his head was a tiny skeleton frame, he was wrapped in pampers, pale, not looking like the Mr. Fabulous we knew but a totally different person.

The preacher told him to ask God and pray that he would be forgiven for his sins and he asked him do you have any last words that you would like to say? With his frail voice, which shook weakly he said to the Minister in his last words. "That is when you want to be a rude boy."

I personally saw the list of the names of all the women that a relative showed to me from the doctors. This list, he told me to hold one end and he would hold on to the other end. We began to roll out that list together, it was four feet long and ten inches wide. People believe me, it contained countless names of women. It was unbelievable, total madness. You can call it what you want, I have never seen anyone who could do such damage to other human beings and this went on for years and years. The relative said to me after all he was my blood but he was a wicked man to women.

Now it was at the same time when I and the relative was speaking about the list, the driver of Mr. Fabulous came and joined us in the conversation, while speaking he told me this list is what we know about of the girls around. He noted that Mr. Fabulous used to go every weekend to all parts of the country picking up girls by the carload, partying with them, then having sex with each one in a hotel before he dropped them home. He went on to say that Mr. Fabulous had been hiring him for years, and there were girls from East, West, North and South of the country that he played himself with.

Now this was apart from what I knew, but I really didn't want to know anymore about it. To be honest this was one individual only and you can see how this went on in a circle and beyond. This clearly shows that one person can give thirty persons in a space of one month the virus, then thirty persons can get it from separate persons in one year's time.

The story of how Mr. Fabulous contracted the HIV virus was a few years prior. He was on the hunt, looking for an apartment to rent and live. He came into contact with a lady who had one upstairs and downstairs house in the area. Whatever the arrangements was, he got through with the lady and the room for rent. He moved into the place, the lady lived upstairs while he stayed in the downstairs apartment.

A couple of days later after, someone in the said area stopped him on the road and made it their business to tell him. "Mr. Fabulous all what you do there, just pay the woman rent and have nothing to do with her."

"Why?" He asked.

The man replied to Mr. Fabulous, "because this lady husband died as a result of AIDS."

Mr. Fabulous said okay, as if it was nothing and paid him no mind. He was warned before renting the apartment too, but as time passed by, months after he was seen coming out from the upstairs house early one morning. This clearly showed that he was having a relationship with the land-lady.

Mr. Fabulous used to sneak in and out from the upstairs house, trying hard for anyone not to see him in the act. This went on for some time, then he got brave enough by going up in the day to this woman.

He became, don't care, maybe he thought people in the area was lying on his land-lady so he was showing the neighbourhood that this woman had no HIV. He started living upstairs common-law and was seen to be very happy in the relationship which went on for some years. Suddenly things changed when the woman became sick. Mr. Fabulous went with her to the doctor knowing what to expect and what the outcome might be. The results was that she was HIV positive, he became startled at first, but since he already built his mind for the moment he remained calm and collected.

They were back to a normal life-style, things were good for the both of them until some time, within a year of the diagnosis that the landlady became very ill. He called the ambulance for her and she was whisked away to the hospital. The doctors did attend to her but when the neighbours visited her she was on drips and very weak in body, she was diagnosed by the doctors with AIDS at this stage. They noted that she would die from any opportunistic infections, some sort of a bad cold or anything.

When this situation arose the neighbourhood had all eyes on Mr. Fabulous, he continued his stay at that house, for how long I couldn't recall but his landlady did pass away as a result of AIDS.

Now this is where he became invisible by hiding indoors for days, no one could see him. Mr. Fabulous was ashamed of people in the area looking at the house night and day. They knew what had happened and that he might be next. It was one cold late night that he went to organize transport, some persons helped him pack everything unto a truck. He quietly moved out of the area where no one could see him and thereon he began his unfaithful, dishonest, hateful, wicked kind of un-love revenge on females- girls who were 16, 17, 18, 19, 20 to 35 years old; single women - women who lived common-law with their man, and countless married women.

From his time then, to those who slept with him then and are still alive today, taking treatment and may continue to sleep with others on and around the country today. Please be careful what you wish for was a reminder, if you are foolish or wise you can either contract the HIV virus or AIDS by buying it or getting it all for free. If you can read and understand you'll know that this thing never stops, it lives on and on, continuing to survive through our blood stream in the veins of us human beings.

However, these blood cells can not take control or survive unless there is sexual penetration or a blood transfusion, it can be also through needles but don't be fooled. Know what is safe sex? Is there really anything today with a partner as safe sex?

Who can you trust but God. **"**

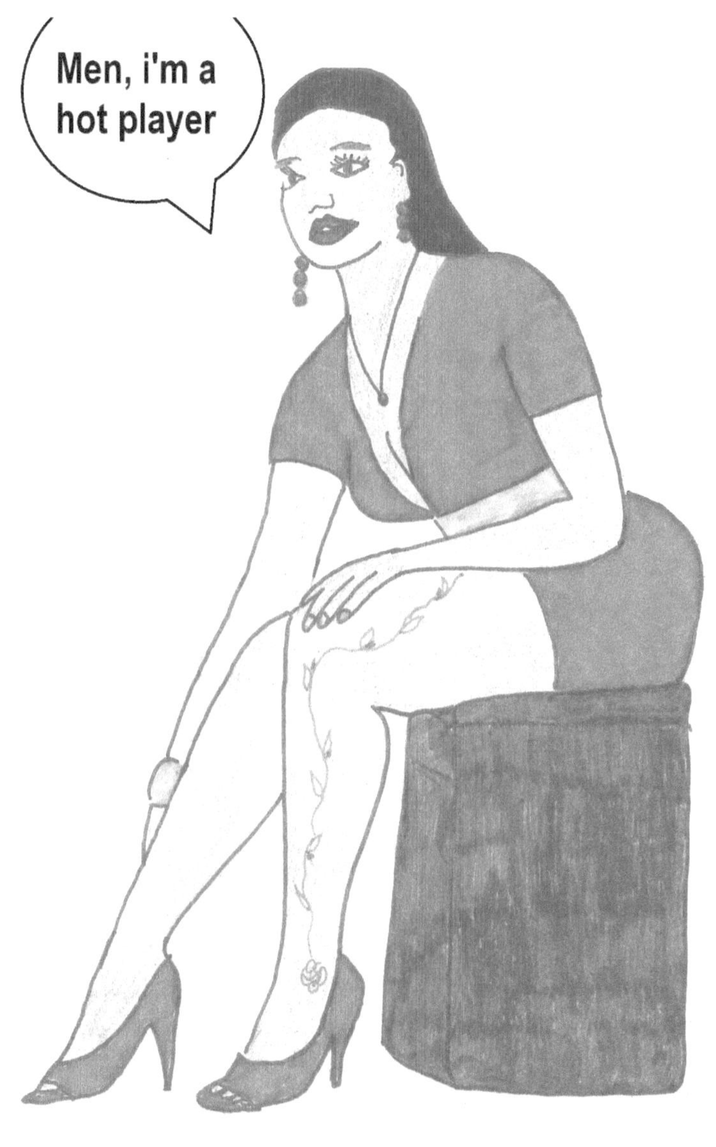
Men, i'm a
hot player

The Plumber

"Of course when coming to plumbing you may think of a vise grip pliers, long and short shovels or a sledge hammer to name a few.

In this story I am going to discuss a plumber, he was a very good work man and a professional at what he did, he was roughly around fifty years old at the time. He was living with his common-law wife and son aged ten, things was nice with both parties for more than ten years. On mornings Plumber would take their son to school before going to work, while mommy stayed at home doing most of the house cleaning. Likewise Plumber would do the same next day, it was very good family living, happiness and togetherness. They had their struggles of life ups and downs just like everyone else, sometimes work would be on a go slow period where Plumber would be at home in between jobs.

Some women, when a man not working often is bacchanal and conflict arising between the two bringing the good relationship to an end. So it was with Plumber, after separating his madam took their son leaving him a lonely man to fend for himself.
He always said, "She's impatient and historically women never satisfied with the little men have but I tried my best as a man to make ends meet, what yuh go do, such is life and the way it is at times."

As they say, "tradesmen[11] don't suffer for long" and knowing Plumber and his type of work he had lots of customers who had jobs for him. Things started picking up again with lots of phone calls from all over, until he hired work men of his own.

Out of all the jobs he got, one was at my next door neighbour's house. This job was to change all the pipe fittings from the tank to the kitchen area in Mrs. Caroline's house. He spent almost the whole day running pipe, now this woman was a married woman with a husband named Shortman. Shortman was a fisherman, selling fish for a living most times. Shortman was never home, he always working, only studying to make money when he reached home at night his wife would be fast asleep already.

She often complained that she never seeing this man, "As he come is to go again. He never have time for me, only work, work!

While working for Ms. Caroline, Plumber saw her situation and he was lonely as much as she was, so he took the opportunity to friend[12] with the man's wife. He often found work to do around

---

11 *Self employed man who works in the construction industry*
12 *Have sex with*

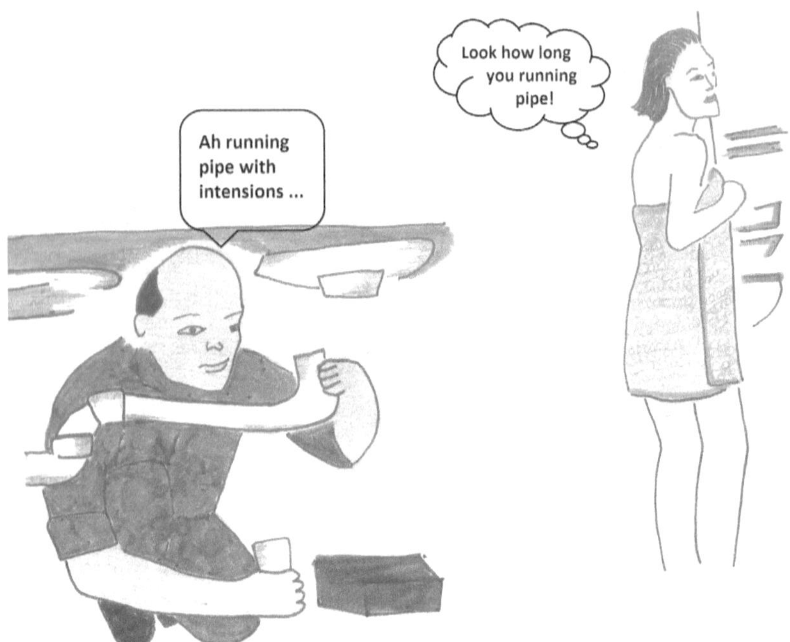

the yard when in fact there was none. They both built a friendship that grew strong, it continued down the road and Mrs. Caroline was now his stand-by lover.

Plumber was the bread winner at the time he and his common law wife was together and she still depended on him for money to get things for her son. He didn't know that when she left him, she already had a man to replace him. She had known the other gentlemen for a while, but what she didn't know is that the man's wife died of AIDS. Regardless of the situation, she went and live with this man for some years well. While living with this man, she knew he was married before and that his wife died from what? He never told her anything or even try to explain why and how, all he kept on saying his wife died years ago and leave him a lonely man until she came into the picture.

You see it's a normal thing and when living in a neighbourhood word does spread on the streets. Knowing she would hear from someone about his wife, that when and how she died, he still didn't tell her. When she heard exactly how his wife died, she confronted him with the situation, it played on her mind for a long time, but she was already in the relationship. So she stayed with him in spite of it all. It was no surprise to her when his condition deteriorated due to his HIV/AIDS status. Some years aback after he became sick at home, she made a phone call for an ambulance to take him to the hospital. I can't recall how long he stayed in the hospital but he stayed critical on drips and medication. I don't know how long he lasted but he died from the disease.

As a man around we knew Plumber very well, so upon hearing the news my mother and I make it our duty to visit him and let him know that his child mother man, who she was living with died as a result of AIDS.

"When this woman comes for money for your son please just give her the money and have nothing to do with her," we advised.

"I does work hard for my money," he answered. "She not getting my money so easy, she have to lie down for it, that is the only way she getting my money."

We said, okay sir have a nice day and left.

There was another friend of mine who also knew Plumber, he is well known for digging graves and burying people in the cemetery. When he heard the news that the child mother man died as a result of AIDS he went by Plumber warning him of this said situation. He pleaded with him: "When your child mother comes for money, it's for your son. For the sake of your own son, just give it to she."

Again Plumber insisted: "No, I does work too hard for my money she have to lie down for it."

His friend turned and explained to him; they were not far from the cemetery, he said to Plumber. "You see that wall next to the cemetery over there?"

Plumber replied yes.

"I am going to bury you right there," his friend declared.

Plumber smiled at him, taking it as a joke.

After all this advice Plumber continued what he was doing by having sex with his child mother in exchange for money and then back and forth dealing with Mrs. Caroline, which is the fisherman's wife. Both women were involved with Plumber at the same time.

When people playing games and fooling around somehow this does never last and it will catch up with anyone of us. When this happens it is going to hunt you until you live to regret life. Nothing lasts forever, Plumber started feeling sick and getting weak with severe headaches that was unbearable for him so he was admitted to the hospital. There doctors told him he would not be able to work anymore because of his condition. Some people get drawn down faster than others, depending on the stages and type of HIV/AIDS. He spent most of his time in the hospital very sick, with just a few months of sickness Plumber's face was already sucking in, all his eyes bulging out of his head. He was not in a good condition he was a very slim person to begin with, when you thin and you don't have much flesh on your body you dry up very fast.

Here now was my plumber friend, shrinking, lying down, he couldn't even move his head or legs. This is life, it so happens his friend who begged him to leave the woman alone visited him in the hospital, sitting at his bedside his friend reminded him of their conversation.

While writing here, I know this is not supposed to be a joke but I can't help but think of the expression, who doh hear, does feel.

I shake my head and laugh at Plumber who was now telling his friend: "Boy if ah did know, ah would have listened to you."

"Ah talk to you, over and over again and others speak to you but you did not want to hear them," his friend cried.

Jack be nimble, Jack be quick, Jack jump over the candle stick. However, Plumber died a couple of months after and he got the promise his friend made him, he dug his hole right next to that cemetery wall, where he was laid to rest and did not have to worry any longer.

His child mother died soon after, I can't say how long but she was laid to rest too. The married woman Mrs. Caroline's husband, Shortman also died as a result of AIDS, which she contracted from Plumber and passed to him.

Shortman died leaving his wife behind. She is still alive today. "

Abie and Ron

alyuh come in
one by one
Ah thirsty
now
ah like it raw
jus so!
alyuh brave
boy!
alyuh have
condoms
boy?

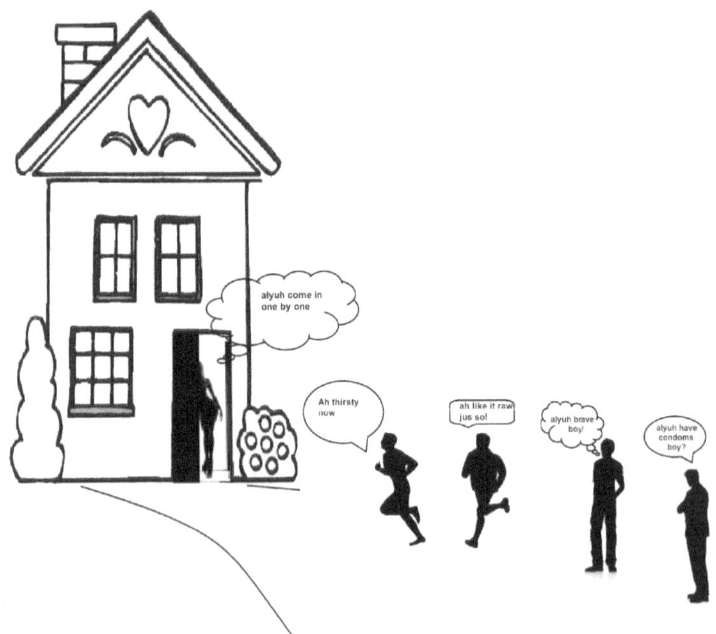

"My neighbour Abie was a close friend to my sister and I, she grew up with her father Norman, who played the role of both mother and father. Abie never knew her mother because she died when she was just five years old. Abie grew up to be a fine, pretty young lady, at nineteen she met Ron, they started dating and after a few months she was pregnant. They both lived in the downstairs apartment of her father's house. They lived a very good life and today their son is 28 years old. Again there were some ups and downs like any relationship but they eventually separated.

Ron left and Abie stayed at home alone with her son.

I really do not know what made Abie do what she did, everyone sometimes get a bit lonely in life but we need to be careful for what we may ask for. It was right next door to me late one night, so I knew. It was not any of my business but I knew what happened. I saw a man knock on Abie's door, she came out and the man went inside with the door remaining open. This one man was having sex with Abie inside, that was clear but on the outside there were ten men from the area lining up, one behind the other thirsty to get their turn to have sex with Abie. I watched this event in amazement to the finish, it seemed none of them used a condom, they all had fun that night.

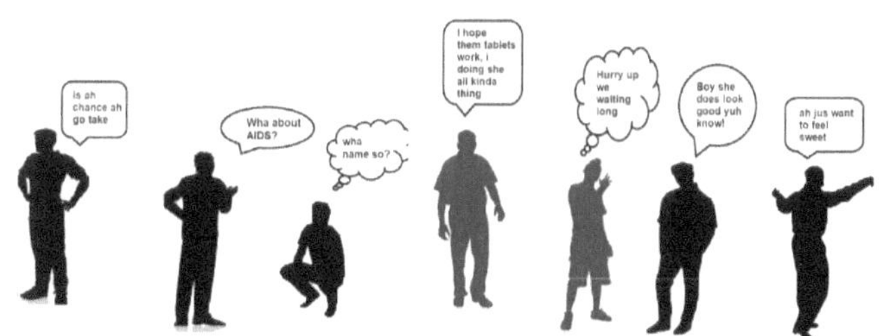

It was about a year or two after that Abie felt ill but she ignored it. I clearly remembered she would go shopping in the nearby mall, not too far from where she lived, while shopping and choosing out a top or skirt in the store she would have a dry cough.

This cough was constant, sometimes it made a sound all the way down her chest. When I asked her why she didn't drink some kind of medication for it, she would reply that it was "small thing, everything normal," even though she had this cough for a while.

A few months down the road she began to take sick at home, this is when we called the ambulance. She was taken to the hospital where an HIV test was done and she was HIV positive. When the news came back to the neighbours that she was taken to the hospital. They wanted to know what was wrong with Abie. As usual the doctors asked who gave it to her and she said she couldn't remember. All I remember is taking eleven men, one after the other so I don't remember who give it to me. However she did give the names of all the men she had sex with for them to get tested. Each one of these men then scratched their head, and most of them moved out of the area due to the situation.

One evening while liming[13] in Norman's make shift park that was built by her father, to my surprise who could I see, but Ron, Abie's child father. After all that time spent away from both of them he returned and we talked.

"What you doing here?" I asked.

"Boy, I come to drop money for my son," Ron replied.

---

13 *Relaxing somewhere doing nothing much*

"Sure but are you aware of the condition of your child's mother," I probed.

"Yes," Ron said.

He admitted that he was aware of her illness but they never stopped seeing each other, when he dropped money, he slept over and left the next morning. I learned that they were still having unprotected sex together.

Abie lasted for more than two years until she became sick and helpless. She was taken to the hospital where they could do no more for her, she eventually passed away with complications due to the AIDS infection.

Ron went on and tried living his life with his son, he was a handy man doing odd jobs while working here and there. From time to time he fell down in the street, an ambulance would come and pick him up and soon he was hospitalized, he tested positive for HIV, which he got from his ex-common-law wife Abie.

Ron is a mystery, although his girlfriend and child mother was sick and he knew what she did with all those men he still resumed the relationship. Maybe for the sake of his son or for love.

With treatment Ron is still okay today. "

Boy Childish

"This story is about a woman named Candybabe, she was a very hard working single mother, with four girls and three boys, seven children.

How did she end up being a single mother of all these children? Well her common law husband and father of every one of those children walked out on Candybabe for a younger woman, he never looked back. From ever since I knew Candybabe she did all types of odd jobs, anything and anywhere to make a dollar to feed her children. I think she did a very good job dealing with all seven children as they grew into big men and women.

Boy Childish was one of her younger sons, he had a girl friend named Stacy for many years but they did not live under the same roof. She used to come and go, I must say they loved each other very much, since they were always hugging real tight, not even breeze could pass through the two of them when they were ready.

Everyone in the area knew Stacey including his family but he didn't like the fact that she came and went occasionally. He was not satisfied with that relationship and chose to move on with his life and got himself a new girlfriend, but as life would have it, Boy Childish did not break up with Stacey.

This man would go out every weekend, Saturday and Sunday to an unknown location in the country, this continued a couple of months well before his mother found out. You see secret don't stay for long and seeing the type of jobs his mother did, cleaning houses and so on. Candybabe happen to be working on a project in the said area, while walking to work there were some men sitting on the block liming.

One of the men asked: "You Boy Childish mother?"

"Yes," she answered.

"Lady talk to your son because that girl who he visiting here is no good girl she is a bad red woman," the man insisted. "It had a man that she was with and he died from AIDS.

Why she come up here to live is because every body know about she from the next area. Talk to your son please."

Upon reaching home Candybabe pulled him square and started questioning him.

"What happened to you and Stacey? What is going on? Who is this new girl friend I am hearing about?" She probed.

"Ma, ah done with Stacey," he answered.

"Yes, but Stacey not done with you," she reminded him. "And

these fellas and them telling me down which part I working that some red girl you pick up and she bad, and one man already died because she give him HIV/AIDS."
"Ma doh study them," Boy Childish replied. "She is a new girl in the area and them jealous me just because they can't have she ma."

Candybabe tried, but to no avail he would listen to his mother but who don't hear does feel. As them old people know it to be, things does be nice all the time until. The following weekend meh boy dress down, gone by the reds only to find she gone back south.

Then he started worrying as to why she would leave him and go, why now? The block boys said to him go get tested for HIV, cause you don't know and this is the reason why we was trying to talk to you all along.

To make a long story short, one and a half years after he started feeling sick suddenly, falling down all over the place, he never did check himself.

He was in and out of the hospital, one evening his mother and I were speaking when we looked up Boy Childish was walking up to where we were standing.

"How are you going son?" She asked.

"Not good girl, not good and ah doh think ah go make it nah," he admitted.

"Ah talk to yuh hard and ah talk to you soft," his mother said. "Ah even cry tears and you not hearing. I tried hard, it have nothing ah could do again."

The following day his mother call the ambulance, they came and carried him to the hospital were he remained warded. He never returned home and died as a result of the HIV/AIDS. His former girlfriend Stacey died about three to four years after, because even though they were separated in between they were having casual sex hence the reason she contracted the HIV/AIDS virus from him.

So when you done, you done. Stay done. Doh make back."

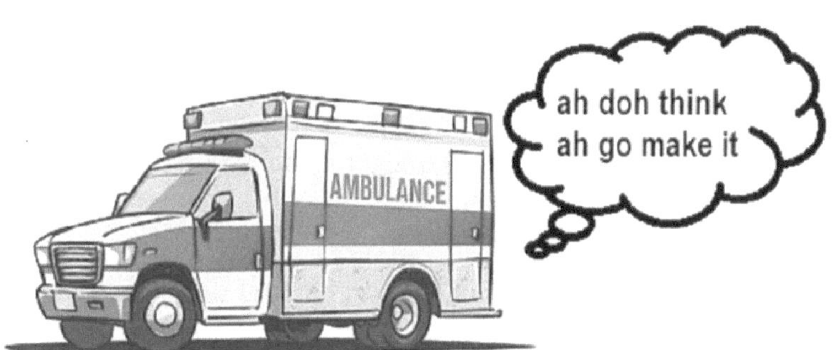

Popo Darlin

"Popo Darlin was a good friend of Mr. Fabulous, both of them used to lime, drink together, hang out in bars. Where ever you see Mr. Fabulous you see Popo Darlin and where ever you see Popo Darlin you see Mr. Fabulous.

Popo Darlin was Mr. Fabulous' riding padner in crime for many years. Popo Darlin was more of a gentleman than his friend, he used to be a real soul man in those days, not too bad looking with a dark complexion.

He was not known to be a games player, most of the times he kept to himself with a cigarette in one hand and a drink in the other. He was a male nurse, which was a good job, I hadn't seen him since the death of Mr. Fabulous. A few years back in some part of the country we both manage to bounce up together in a venue.

He noted that we needed to talk, I agreed but I didn't know what the conversation would be about. We found a spot, sat down and began to chat. While listening to what he had to say, I realized that it was not about Mr. Fabulous but about his personal life which was interesting to hear. He went on to say that at his work place there was a girl who had been admiring him for a long time but he paid no attention to her because she was his co-worker.

"So what is your real problem?" I asked.

He admitted that dating a co-worker was out of the question, and they were like family working together as a team for years and years, but she was persistent. She even followed the man to the toilet, going in the Cafeteria behind him in at lunch hour, she was with him every afternoon at home time.

So Popo Darlin tell himself he would give her a try and see where it goes.
She invited him out on a dinner date and promised to pay all expenses. Meh boy say he take that offer with a smile and both of them went out and had a nice time, his head was bad from drinking rum and other alcohol and he brought her home with him because she said it was too late for her to go home.

He said they started kissing from outside until they reach the bedroom, then clothes began to fly all over, he was inside it in a split of a second and was action all night until morning.

With all he telling me the big question remained, "Popo Darlin, you use a condom?"

"No boy," he said, "You mad, no rubbers with that girl."

"But Popo you see what happen to your padner and you eh learn nothing," I chastised him.

He went on to say a few months after he was feeling sick and would fall down on the job, sometimes he would knock-out cold not knowing a thing that happened.

The doctors decide to run some tests on their co-worker and he was HIV positive. He did explain to the doctor that he never had the disease before and that he was a careful man and the only person he had sex with recently was their co-worker. She was called upon to take the test and she was HIV positive.

He told me a meeting was held forthwith and they made a decision to transfer her out to another location.

Popo Darlin was not happy, I said to him that it already happen so just live. He however admitted he had another girl friend who was living with him but before they meet she was already HIV Positive. He told me that they were going to keep the germs between the both of them.

Popo Darlin is alive today, as I write, he is continuing to take treatment and at the end of our conversation, he said that he will keep to himself and his girl and would not do what his friend Mr. Fabulous did to other women. **"**

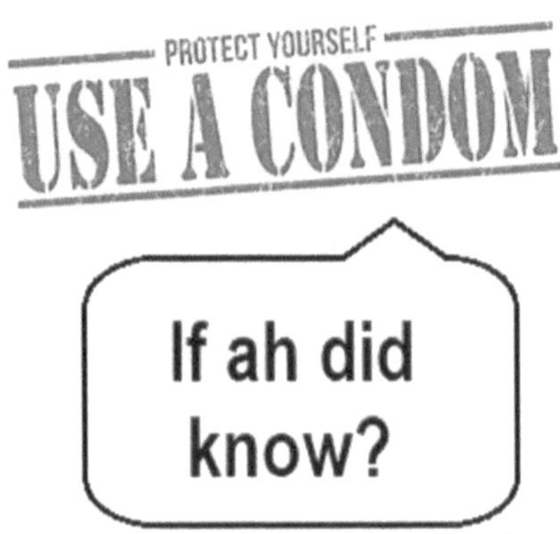

Jim the Piper

A Piper is a drug addict who sells everything to buy drugs

"It was the year 1996 to be exact. Jim was a working class person who properly attired himself whether at home or at work. He was a sprightly young, dark handsome fellow who came from a large family of fourteen to maybe seventeen children.

His was a known family to me and others, we were very close friends with each other, whenever he got to go out meh boy used to make it his duty to come and drink with me. He would carry on many long boring conversations, then I did not see him again for weeks. I did not see him again until he appeared in my shop with huge boxes of records for me to conduct sales for him to get money.

It seemed that Jim was in a desperate money position at times. These records were LP's and 45's by the hundreds, lots of oldies music. So I put them on display for him, so anyone who walked by my shop could see them and make a purchase. This kind of stock really stayed on my hand for a while but I made sure and got every one sold. Every time I called Jim, he would just grab the money out of my hand and leave in a rush. Then I would wonder what was going on with this man, I thought he was on some kind of drugs or something because he wasn't moving right at all.

I also noticed that when we spoke he developed a way of bowing down over my counter top, just so.

"What's wrong with you?" I would ask. "Is there a problem?"

"Boy ah feeling tired, ah weak and I need to buy tablets?" He would reply.

"For what?" I wanted to know but he never answered me.

It was not even a few days after that he started bringing anything he got his hands on to sell, this was the remaining items, things like a turn-table. He said he had nothing to play on it, so why keep It and other parts of his music system: his amplifier, equalizer, speaker boxes, all was old. Then he brought household items pots, pans, and even dishes into my shop. I told him none of that, just carry those things back home. This went on for a period of time then I stopped seeing him again.

It was his brother who came one day and said to me. "Boy you know Jim flat out and could not move his legs or arms but was just in bed lying down."

His brother noted that Jim asked him for water and asked him to help him up, which he did after giving him the cup of water. Jim passed away in his brother's arms, his last words to this brother was.

"Boy ah going."

His brother asked, "Yuh going?"

And he replied, "Yeah ah going."

Jim passed away, he was really small in body and weighted less than a fifty pound bag of flour.

Jim confessed to his brother that he used to run girls, good girls then he made a wrong choice. Jim was a working class person but he used to find himself going to the market places everyday and night after work to buy weed and cocaine. The drugs lead him to have unprotected sex with piper girls who were also on drugs which gave him the HIV virus. This was making him sick all along and he was hiding it from his friends and family.

This is why Jim died so soon, too soon.**"**

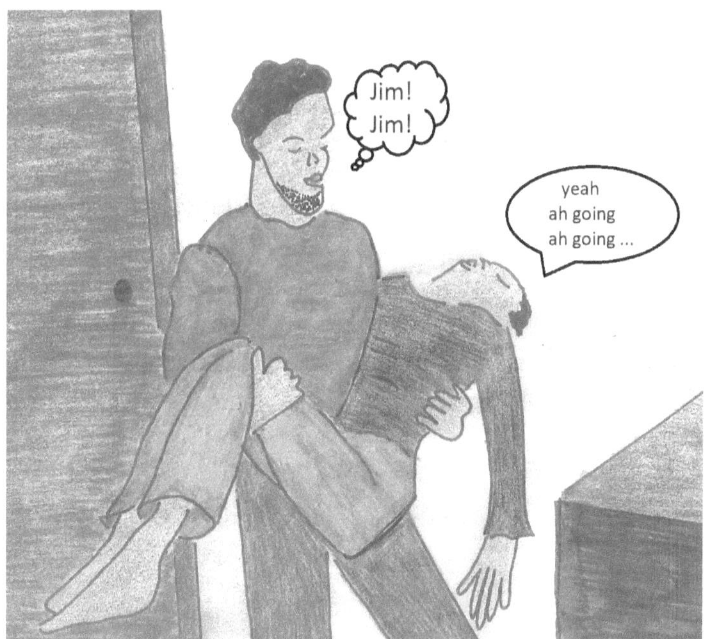

Bun Bread Hustler

"This is a similar story to the one of Jim, the first time I meet Bun Bread, he was in the corridor just a step away from my shop door. He said good morning to me and I said good morning, what can I do for you sir?

There our conversation began, he was a kind-hearted man, friendly and talkative. His story is my shortest, within a year or less of meeting him, while we sat and talked, I notice the top and bottom of his lips were peeling. They were cracked up badly, each time he came to the shop it got worst, when I asked him what's wrong with your lips. He would say he needed some hops to go home with and burn them and put all together in a mug to make a thing he called cooling water because his body was too heated.

"It heated, meh body heated okay," he would say every time.

I didn't argue.

He was unemployed when he borrow money from me to buy the bag of hops bread. It wasn't every day he would pass but occasionally whenever he passed is toaster oven and almost any mini appliance he selling me.

Then my question would be, "Why you selling out your stuff and what will you use when everything done?"

He would say I need the money for medication purposes my health is at risk, but he never said what the health risk was or why he continue to do what he was doing until every thing was gone.

After that I did not see nor hear anything from him for a long while.

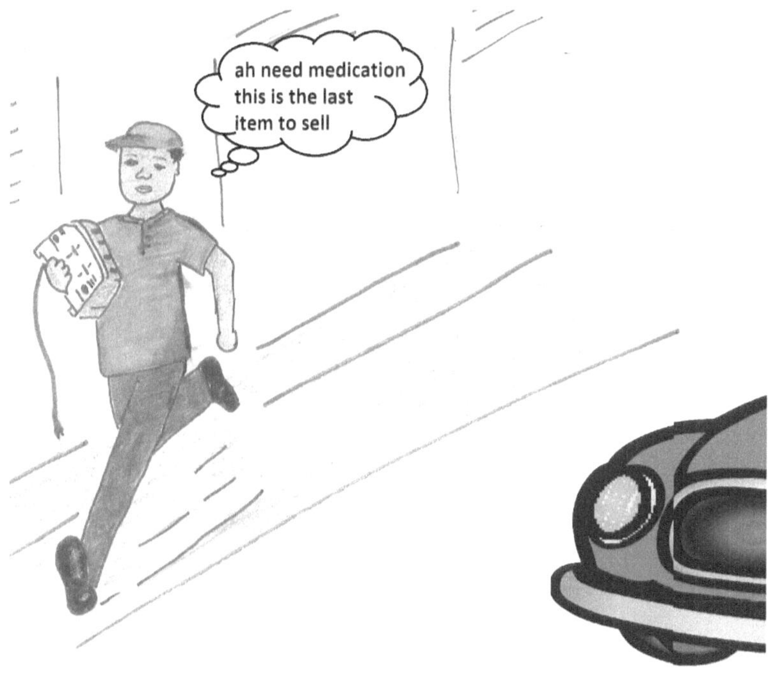

Maybe a year after, early in the morning while walking through the streets a mister shout out my name from across the road. When I went to meet that person, he asked me if I remembered my friend, the man who used to lime inside the shop.

I noted there were many people, lots of them come into my shop. It's then he said the man with all the mini appliances, that I bought from him.

Yes, I remembered Bun Bread and asked what happened to him. "Boy, the man dead," was his reply.

I was surprised and asked from what.

"Mr. AIDS," the man said.

I wondered how long he had it and the man explained that Bun Bread had HIV for over five years. This was the reason he was sick and it was also the reason why he was selling out everything because he was so sick.

People with their foolish and silly ways, sickness can happen to anyone of us but there are treatments for it.

There are many people living with HIV/AIDS today and they don't feel ashamed, you can live a normal life. I wish some people knew that.**"**

One Man Leather

"In my neighbourhood, there lived a family member who was a good craftsman. He could make anything for man, woman or child.

One Man Leather was a nice person, very respectful, down to earth and friendly to his customers. He was so good with his craft that other craft-men would visit him to learn new ideas that he would share, even foreigners made orders with this man.

Nevertheless, he was hardened, ignorant and hard of hearing towards his girlfriend. They both ran the business together, and his workload was so heavy that they would usually carry items home, to work on for the next day. This was a good and honest business, which they did together for over five years but their business came first.

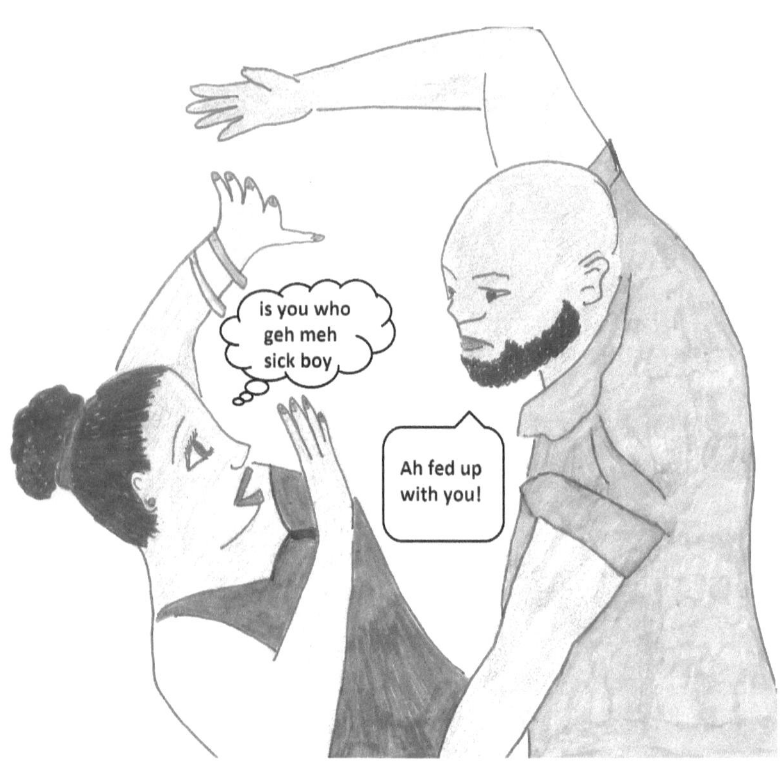

One day his girlfriend decided to end the relationship, I can't say what happened but she packed her clothes and other stuff and moved out leaving him and his business.

One Man became lonely but after a short period he got involved with a much younger woman who had a child, they both moved in with him.

Things started off good between them, it was business as usual again, she would go open up the shop while he dropped her son to school. He built a good relationship with his new step-son since he never had children of his own.

These two lived together well above two years but one night we heard quarrelling among them, it was a heated argument, she kept saying, "Since I with you, ah feeling sick, weak and tired, just so. You better hope I doh have nothing cause ah never was sick, meh son depend on me and is he ah living for!"

The next day she ups and visit the doctor for a check up only to find out that she was HIV infected. Upon reaching back home there was more quarrelling until it turn into fighting, neighbours all around intervened and tried to separate them.

Things eventually came to a calm as she declared, "You better get ah test if you know what good for you."

Soon he too left for a visit to the doctor, when all the check up was done he was HIV positive but it seems that he had it for a long while.

The doctor asked him, "How many women you slept with?"

"Only two," he answered surprised. Which was his last girlfriend and the one he had now.
He went straight to the first girl-friend home. He knocked on the door but there was no answer.

"One Man, who are you looking for?" The neighbour next door asked.

"My ex," he told the neighbour.
"Boy, she died a while now, and the man she was living with he died too," the neighbour confirmed.

"From what and how?" One Man asked

"HIV AIDS" the neighbour said. "AIDS"

One man wasted no time, in a haste he headed for home. He tried putting his girl friend to sit down, tried explaining to her that he didn't know, tried telling her what happened and that he was sorry for what had been done.

At that stage she didn't want to hear anything from him, she thought him to be a mad man asking her to forgive him, due to the circumstances she took her son and left.

The following year he fell ill and was bed-ridden, he had stayed too long before getting treatment and died as a result of the HIV/AIDS virus. His last girlfriend also died years after from complications of the virus."

Zesty the Hitman

"Zesty was a man of wealth, power and strength. He was big, black, strong, muscular and intimidating looking. He was born with a cokey eye[14] so when you feel he was watching you, is someone or somewhere else he was looking at. He lived with his wife and children in a large mansion, he wanted for nothing maybe only to find Jesus Christ.

Most of his time was spent travelling to the United States of America, he went almost three times each year. Whenever he was back in the country, he worked his car as a taxi in his spare time. On my way to work, I might be in luck to travel with him and then we would talk about almost anything that comes to mind.

While speaking I never asked him his business, he was the one who brought up these personal issues about himself so I listened attentively.

---

14 *Lazy eye*

"Boy, I have to talk to somebody," Zesty started.

"When ah use to travel in the earlies together with a friend we will go to New York for three to six months, and that was not to work or do any kind of business transaction whatsoever."

So I started wondering what this man going to tell me here. Then he said he and the same friend would go and run down white girls, who looking nice, with good shape and they would pay money in US dollars to have great sexual intercourse with them.

"Sir, you were working," I joked.

It sounded like a joke then but this was how he was making his money all those years gone by. After those conversations about his other life, I did not see him for over a year or more.

However, after one time is the next so sooner or later he was back and working his car on the road again. I did not make him out at first, because he was driving a brand new vehicle. It was only when he stopped that I realized it was him.

"How are you and how have you been keeping?" I asked happily.

"Not in good shape," he admitted, I wasn't sure if he was watching me or the door.

"But you are big and strong sir," I responded.

"Not in that way I mean," he answered.

"And how is that?" I asked him.

"Boy ah does go New York and spend time, why you don't see me so," he continued not saying much.

"What about that friend of yours? I cyah tell the last time ah see him either," I probed.

In a sad and withdrawn face Zesty admitted to me that all of them who went to be with women, he and his padner included contracted the HIV virus. When I asked him if he remembered which one of the girls give the disease to him and his friend, he couldn't say.

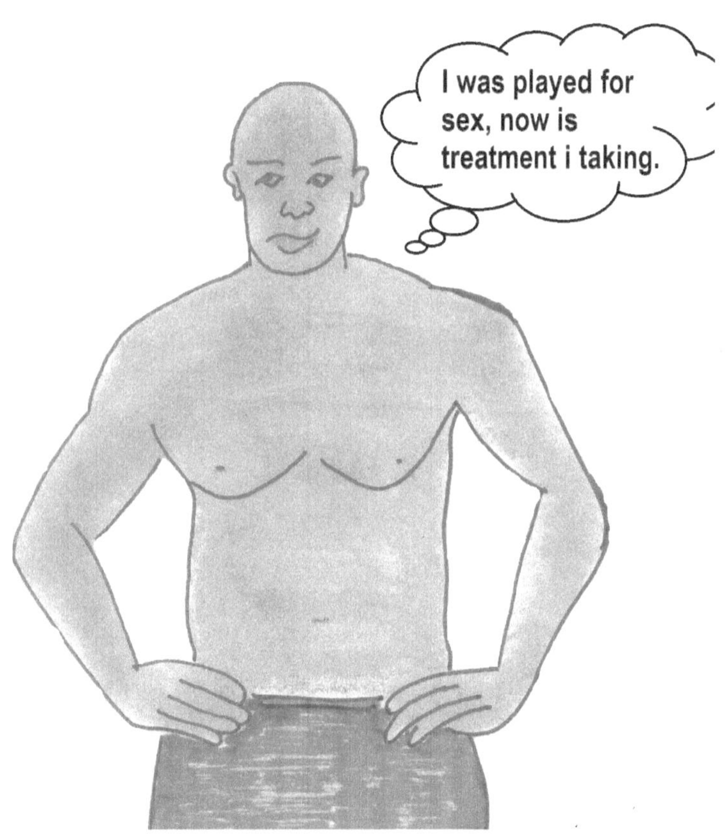

"Ah really doh know, is hundreds of girls we had sex with over the years, hundreds," Zesty said. "Look how things does be, now I travelling for treatment because I sick from fooling around."

As time went by his wife fell ill, not knowing what was taking place she told him she needed some space and went back home by her mother where she later died from complications of the virus.
This made Zesty real lonely, not long after the next door neighbour who knew well that his wife died from HIV and that he was sick with HIV, went and married Zesty for his money.

He died soon after he couldn't battle with the deadly disease anymore, however his new wife ended up with all his money and most of all his HIV virus. **"**

Mama Jah and Papa Jah

"This story is about two people Mama and Papa Jah, husband and wife. They bought an unfinished property in the neighbourhood and moved in with their children. All of them was accommodated in the downstairs apartment only. In those days, I looked at Mama Jah as a contented woman because she made do with little and made things work.

After a year they stared constructing the upper part of the house, it was completed in a matter of months. Pap Jah was a financier in the neighbourhood, his customers would borrow from him and pay back through the bank as to avoid bad paying persons.

Mama and Papa Jah lived happy together for thirty-three years, until Papa Jah started sleeping out and coming home the next day. The large sums of money went to his head, he would leave for days, then weeks which turned into months. Soon he was gone for years and then just never came back.

So they were separated. In the beginning Mama Jah knew something was not right, then she found out about the outside women. He was sleeping around almost anywhere he could because he had plenty money with big interest coming in.

Mama Jah moved on just as he did, she found herself a good boy-friend. It helped with the loneliness but not the way she wanted because she really loved her husband. She turned to alcohol, she drank and smoked her frustration away. She was liming in bars in all parts of town. On many occasions whilst I was coming from work on evenings Mama Jah would be sitting on the sidewalk drunk. I used to put her in a taxi, in order to get her safely home. This went on for a while until she became sick from the alcohol consumption, the doctors put her on a diet and stopped her from drinking and smoking. From there she made a big change in her life and began to go to church. She became a Christian and as time passed she began feeling ill again. She visited the doctors who told her that she was sick with her heart and was referred to other doctors for treatment.

A few days after Mama Jah tried getting in contact with her husband. Upon doing so she found out that he was warded at the hospital, he was sick with bronchitis, he had a bad cold of some kind. She paid her husband a visit and found out he was terminally ill with AIDS. For Mama Jah this was no good news for any one but she stood her ground and took care of him. Papa Jah lived for a period of time before succumbing to death by HIV/AIDS. Mama Jah kept on and continued to live a life of God.

After work I would pass by Mama Jah and we would sit and talk, she used to give me very good advice and I never asked her what was ailing her. One day she told me about her heart disease and I respected her. She would be in and out of the hospital frequently and one day she told me that the doctors gave her five days to live.

It was not a good thing to hear at the time, but such is life so I sat with her everyday. God has the last word to say and it was not five days it was less. She told me she had made peace with

God and that she was ready to meet him. These were her last words to me: "Don't worry because Jesus will help you, yes he will help you."

On the following day Mama Jah was gone. She passed away peacefully at the hospital, the funeral arrangements were made and she was laid to rest.

Meanwhile her boyfriend, very soon after her death became sick in an untimely manner, he died after being diagnosed with flown blown AIDS.

Nevertheless the last woman that Papa Jah was living with was still alive, she got a stroke and is now bed-ridden. In his case no one knew how many women he was with over the years and a few of them were right around the area. **"**

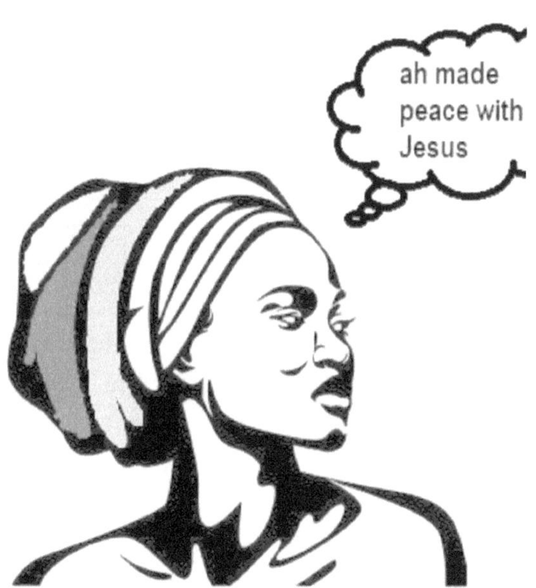

Tobago Love

"As a little boy growing up my father would take us to Tobago by boat probably once every year. We usually stayed by my aunt's hotel which was The Golden Thistle next to Crown Point International Airport at the time.

This was a very nice place back in the days, where most of the Calypsoians like the Mighty Shadow, Calypso Rose, Baron and many other popular names in the Calypso world of music would come to entertain the massive crowd that was there. Most of the guests were foreigners from all over the world. All this was happening just walking distance from the beach area, where people after taking a bath in the sea would come and swim around in the pool. My other aunt would do the cooking, she made a delicious crab and dumpling with callaloo and coconut oil down. There was also a huge bar on the inside with all types of drinks to choose from. In that little surrounding of the hotel there was also a beautiful courtyard with a rental car business. Everything you needed was on that compound.

Most of my time was spent walking on the beach, I loved it, I would walk from one point to the other for hours. While doing so I met a body builder and became familiar with him around the hotel. He liked to lime by the beach, he would watch each and every white woman that passed, he would call out to them and he would get a good response every time. They would come over and chat with him for very long, he was muscular and physically fit, so these girls would hold unto him and rub their hands all over his body.

There was one girl who caught his attention real good but he was not the only man that this white girl had. She was dealing with around fifteen other men besides him. I can not recall what country she was from but she was paying men in US dollars to have sex with her in a hotel while she was staying in Tobago. Now this body builder said this with his own mouth that he would go up to her hotel room, sometimes four and five times to have sex with this white chick because she gave him good US money to do so. She was in her late fifties, but looking dam good, blond with a nice shape.

It happened however that a month or more after that she made a public announcement and was also interviewed by the media that she was HIV positive. She went on to say that the fifteen men and more that went into the hotel room with her knew, she said she told them that she was HIV positive and they still wanted to have sex with her and she paid them in US currency. The media asked: Did any of the men wanted to use condoms? She replied no.

This was thirty years ago. When we visited the Golden Thistle my aunt would always warn us to stay away and be careful of those white girls. At the time I really did not understand what she meant because all I was seeing was nice girls, looking good. While sitting back on one of those chairs around the poolside, relaxing myself, I would all of a sudden see a beautiful white girl in a two piece bathing suit, great shape walking around the pool. She would dive and swim around the pool for a bit then come out and relax on one of the chairs in a compromising position. She would attract everything. Then I would remember my aunt telling me to stay away.

How could I do such a thing when I seeing such a nice woman before me. She was forty-two years old and came to spend three months. All the rooms in the hotel was in a circle around the pool, there was a room where a young man stayed right next to her. After hours when everyone was inside this young man would sneak into her room and come out the next morning. This went on for a month so I tell myself he can't get all that action for himself. I stood there staring at the woman, I tell you this was very tempting for me, to see him getting everything - all that free action - and me nothing.

The next day she was in another bikini, but still I didn't think about what my aunt said to me, I was only watching her. Then I noticed that something was not right that night, she was gone by the next morning. There was no sight of this white lady she was nowhere to be seen. All she left was an envelope at the front desk for my aunt to give to the young man.

My aunt sent me to fetch the man, I found him and told him that my aunt needed to see him.

"For what and why?" He asked

I really did not know the details, all I could explain that he had some letter at the front desk. He came and my aunt gave him the letter.

I was curious and watched him open it, there was six thousand US dollars in that envelope with a short note.

He wondered aloud why she would go and leave him money. He opened the note and read aloud. "Thank you for everything and the good times we had together. I want you to take this money for your funeral arrange-ment because I have AIDS."

My aunt had to call this young man's mother and father to come for him, he could not be-lieve what he had just read.

I am not con-demning all these women who visit-ed back in the days but I think most of them really in-tended to spread the HIV virus among the locals.

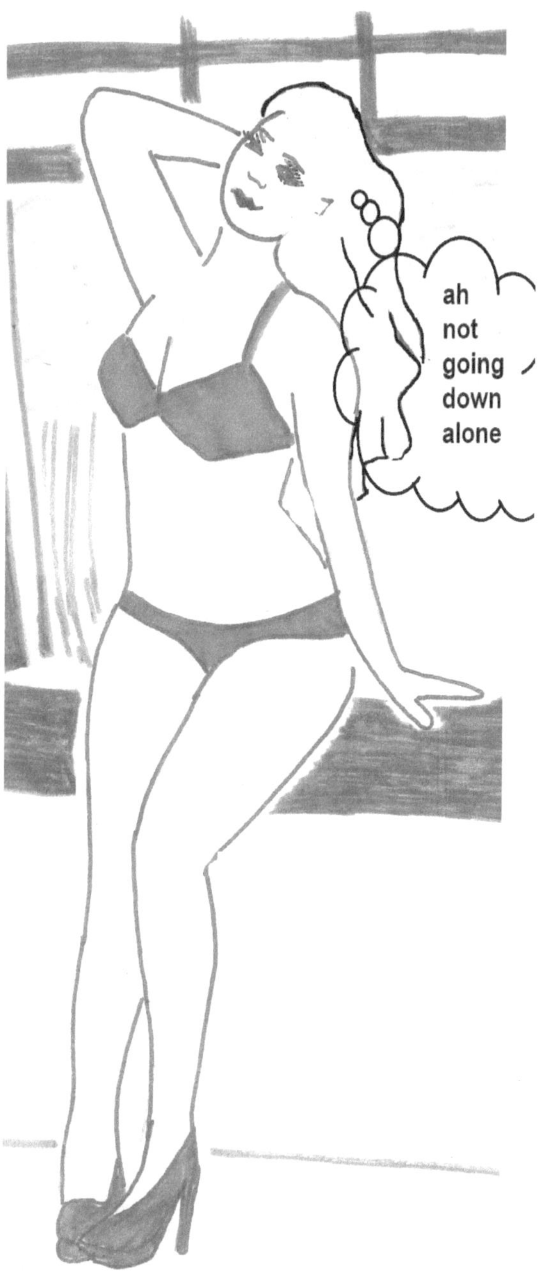

They came, infected and left without looking back. Knowing that some of these men were living with wives and children, it was a sad state back then.

I think that HIV/AIDS may not be as rampant in the world today if it wasn't spread without a thought for life.**"**

HORNING

"Within our culture we usually refer to the act of infidelity as a horn.

Horn or horns is a bony projection pointed in an upwards position on the head of various animals such as sheep, goats, cattle or antelopes.

Sometimes we trini feel that we can out grow any one of these animals horn, which means man or woman while she or he is away from home is ah next man jumping the wall, coming through the back door of the house, heading towards the bedroom, hoping she's undressed and naked under the cover waiting and ready to get things started, playing for time before her husband comes back home. When trinbagoians horn[15] most of the time, one hundred percent it's with someone they are familiar with and of no surprise, not very far away or right next door. You get horn from your wife and you give horn to your wife, these types of horn happen within family members, good friends, best friends, close friends, acquaintances, close relatives, uncles, aunts, brothers, sisters, like every day is horning.

---

15 *To be unfaithful in your relationship*

Nearly Dead Horning

There was an incident that happened a few years ago between two good friends. Real good friends, liming, drinking, cooking, dancing, eating together on weekend but with all that fun, his good friend was watching the man wife all along. As he turned his back is horn for so. So he not only eating ah food from his best friend wife but the food in the pot as well as drinking anything in the refrigerator. He would leave before the husband comes home.

"Is a timing thing with we, and a chance we would take," he would say.

It so happened that one day the husband "made a tack[16] back" only to see his best friend and neighbour with his wife having sex in a compromising position, a position that she had never did with him before. Both men started quarrelling and fighting, a struggle ensued between and the husband took a knife and dealt the man several stabs about his body. The neighbour was badly damaged he was rushed to the hospital and remained unconscious in a critical condition.

16 *Return home unexpectedly*

The husband upon hearing what happened, knowing he nearly killed his best friend left home in frustration. He was afraid and hoped that the man didn't die because it meant police and jail if anything happened to his best friend, not knowing what the outcome may be he went to the agricultural shop and purchased a bottle of weedicide.

He went back home and drank the entire bottle, he was found frothing from the mouth by passing neighbours, who took him to the hospital, so he ended up in a critical condition as well.

Now both these men were in critical conditions, after hours of operation only one of the men survived. This man was the honer-man. He is alive today and is currently living with the man's wife and his daughter comfortable, comfortable in the same house, the dead man's house.

In situations like these it is not the neighbour to lay blame on, if he had an honest, genuine and faithful woman at his side this would not have resulted in the man being stabbed about his body, but he is alive today.

This picture shows that she was the slacker, she was not satisfied with one man and if she can do it to her dead husband then why not the honer-man later down the road with a next man, a new man.

All these situations I think is due to vice.

Vice is in your head, it plays with your emotions. Why will we do these things just to satisfy our ego? Sex is fun with lots of excitement, I am not saying it isn't but that excitement can turn into sadness when you are not being truthful or disease and even death. Death comes by the same man or woman that you were familiar and smiling with.

In our country most of us will say horning each other is part of our culture, and if we don't horn we are not trini's. **"**

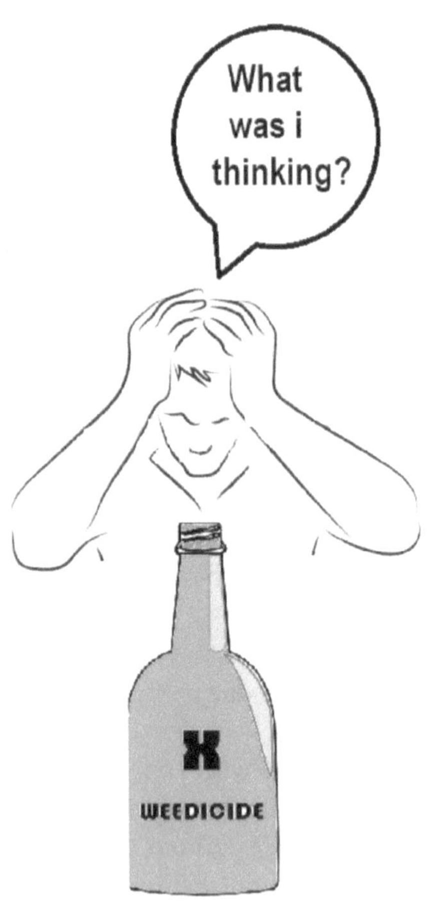

Prim and Pablo

"Apart from the other horn story, I wanted to write this one because it is interesting and I think someone may learn something from reading it.

I don't know how I was able to be on spot for these events when they happened, some say it was luck but most of all it was a great experience for me to write a story, one I never knew would be told. What is life without an experience? Then you wouldn't have a story to tell.

A few years ago in the early 90's, it was the dry season. Early one morning I was walking down the street, on my way to work. I saw a nice dougla[17], a very pretty young lady, she was tall and skinny, as she walked opposite to me I noticed she had sores, lots of sores all over her body but not on her face.

With a very low tone she said" "Good morning sir."

For which I replied. "Good morning to you beautiful and how are you? My name is Robby and what's your name love?" I asked

"Dorn," she answered.

---

17 *Mixed Indian and African heritage woman*

"How may I be of help to you?" I inquired.

"Well I am here in the area looking for an apartment," she divulged. "It's for me and my two children, one boy and one girl."

I really did not know of any empty apartment space for rent in the area but there was a old man by the name of Pablo who I recommended to her. I told her, he may be able to help you get a place for you and those kids, then I went to work.

On my way home, that evening I meet Pablo down the road, I asked him if a girl named Dorn, who was looking for a room came to see him. He told me yes, he already made some arrangements with her for an apartment the following week. Now there was an abandon house with two bedrooms, a dining room and kitchen. It was a flat house just below from where I lived. It was not two good days when four men started cleaning up the whole house inside and outside, all the bush and tall grass was cut down.

When I asked, I found out that Pablo had contacted the owner a day after meeting Dorn and made preparations for this girl because after understanding her situation, how she had no money, no furniture, no groceries and nobody wanted to help her out, without hesitation or doubt Pablo decided to help Dorn out in any way he could.

Pablo paid the first month's rent with one in hand, thinking that she will continue on her own but the next month she still had no money, because she worked nowhere so she drew no pay. Pablo paid another month feeling sorry for this girl he was pursuing. Dorn saw his weakness, that he wanted to help her which was an opportunity for him to be close to her. So he continued to pay rent and buy groceries for her and her two children.

Dorn realized that Pablo was a lonely old man and she herself did not have anyone because of her condition I spoke of before. She had sores all over her body and no man wanted anything to do with her. Pablo told Dorn that he would pay for her to go to a doctor to look at the sores and he would pay for her medical bills and whatever tablets she needed. The next day bright and early they were off to the doctor, they went together, she took a medical exam and it was not HIV it was a form of chicken pox which was curable and not harmful to humans.

She started taking her pills and eating all the proper food that was needed and in a few months this girl started to spread from the hips, bottom putting on size and all the sores disappearing from her skin, it began to look smooth.

When Dorn dress up every one of the men on the block who used to scorn her, who didn't want her from before, who never tried to help her, these same men were now looking at her even tracking her now, because Pablo have her looking so good.

After one thing is another both Pablo and Dorn start to build a relationship together, things was so nice the man was feeling like sixteen again, with this young heart in his life. Then I saw a brand new bed arrive, the next month was freezer and then table with chairs, in the forth month a new washing machine and wardrobe, the fifth month was kitchen cupboards being built by my other neighbour named Prim.

Before you knew it Dorn had everything, that any other woman had just to make her happy and comfortable.

Each and every day she would cook for Pablo and call him down to eat, although they were not living together they had a good relationship, strong and stable.

The men in the area would call out to Dorn when she dressed up sexy and passed them by: "Sexy, sexy dougla, nice girl, you making style on we?"

"Yes," she would say, "because when I did come up here before I meet Pablo, all of you was first and none of you all helped me. Is Pablo who took me in and take good care of me and even put me and my children in house. Now you all calling me, because ah looking good now, ah doh want to hear all yuh. Pablo is my man and de man at the moment and I happy with that."

Pablo was a retired man who worked with the Government. Now and again private contractors would come and take him to do jobs for them twice a week. Now Prim was also my neighbour from next door, he was the carpenter who built the cupboards in the kitchen area.

Dorn and Prim used to talk and they became very close friends, each and every morning Prim would go down and lime with Dorn. I observe this thing and I wondered why Prim going by the man woman, sometimes even Pablo would pass and watch them liming.

One day early, Pablo and I saw each other on the road and as we spoke we noticed that Prim was already by Dorn in the gallery of the house.

Pablo and I looked at each other.
"Pablo watch that wha going on dey?" I said.

"Seeing, ah watching that ah long time now," Pablo answered. Then Pablo shout out, "Dorn! Dorn! Wha he doing dey?"

"So he cah lime with me, you have a problem with that too?"

Dorn shouted back. "Then I can't have no friends Pablo! Pablo if you going down the road go nah, go yuh way."

Pablo told me that he going down the road and would make a tack back to see what was really going on.

I went home, it was not a few good hours yet when I started hearing big bacchanal coming from Dorn's house, only to see Prim running up full speed by my house, leaving Dorn and Pablo quarrelling with each other.

I ask Prim: "What you do to the man girl?"

He told me for himself that he and Dorn grew feelings for each other by talking to each other each day and that he could not help it because she was looking too good to be true. So I ask her for a brush[18] and he went on to say that she never refuse him. They went to one of the bedrooms where Dorn undress herself. She took off every piece of clothes she had on and remained in her bra and panties. He grabbed her and ran into a corner of the room, lifted her off the ground, suspended in the air with her legs spread apart and started banging her against the wall while she ran her fingers through his hair. With a loud voice she shouted: "Prim! Prim! Oh God you sweet Prim. Give meh it, is just so I like it."

Meanwhile Pablo walk into the dinning room, when he heard the commotion he walked into the bedroom where Prim and Dorn was and kicked opened the door. Only to see Prim have his girl, Dorn suspended in the air banging her against the wall of the house.

Pablo stood in shock watching them, he couldn't seem to come to terms with himself until he said: "Yes, is you Prim? Prim my

18 *To have sex*

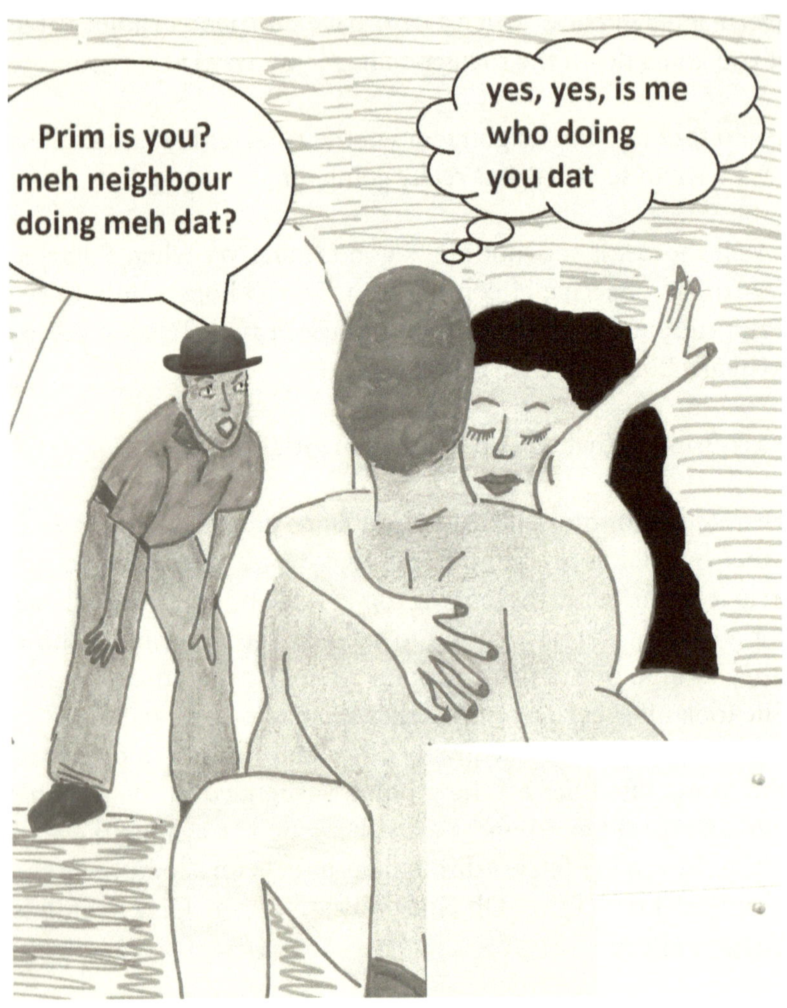

neighbour. Yes? Is you who doing meh that?

Prim said yes.

With disbelief Pablo walked out and went next door in rage to another neighbour.

"Neigbs ah catch them," Pablo declared. "You know ah catch

84

them."

"Pablo who you catch?" The neighbour asked.

"Dorn and Prim brushing," Pablo admitted.

"What you go do now?" She asked him.

"Girl, I don't know, I really don't know," Pablo sighed.

Pablo leave from by the neighbour and went down the road, he watch the stand pipe, open it and watch the water running out of it, then he sat under the running water for almost the rest of the day.

No one, not even his children could talk him out from under that pipe.

It was one week after the bacchanal that Pablo decide to visit Dorn face to face by force. In doing so he level with her by saying: "Dorn I hurting inside, I can't eat, I can't sleep. Why you do meh that? What you did with my neighbour Prim was totally disrespectful to me, after all we've been through and everything that I did for you, this is what I get in return?"

"But Pablo you know I love you," Dorn lied.

"You call that love?" Pablo asked.

"Well Pablo shit does happen and I am a young woman," Dorn replied. "I like plenty of sex and you is ah old man. How much you could do to satisfy me, that's why I take Prim and he doing it better than you."

"Dorn, no more," Pablo begged. "I don't want to hear any more and I done with you . I am not responsible for you and your children any more. Just take them things and go."

So Dorn came with nothing and left with two truck load of furniture and appliances.

However, Dorn and Prim continued their relationship, until they got married for some years. Prim got in an accident and his neck was broken, today his wife Dorn is now going to church and serving God.

Unto this day, Pablo remained a lonely old man at 86 years old.

When you play with fire you does get burn.**"**

Pat and the Iron Man

"This story starred a husband and wife who lived together with their three girls and one boy, at one time everything was good, and everyone was happy until Mr. Horn came into play.

Now many men in the country, I believe have experienced the word horn in real terms, but knowing our Trinidadian men who sometimes call themselves macho. A macho man have plenty pride, so even though it happen to them they will try to keep it a secret. I have known lots of men all my life who this happened to until I was like an adviser or even a full time councillor for hours at times, for days and weeks trying to bring some sort of comfort in their lives.

As for me, I never took a course in counselling or in any other area, my schooling was just on the secondary level but all that was done for these people worked fine for me. These types of problems were very technical ones to deal with because situations like these can results in killings or wounding with intent. These situations may separate family members, it may even break them apart or put them back together, it depends on what you advise and how you advise the matter to be handled.

Let me continue with this couple, although there are so many, too many I have seen, if I try to write them all this book will never end.

At one point my next door friend was a tradesman better known as Iron Man. He went to work each day just to make sure his family was okay, to bring food to the table and put money in his wife pocket which was the happiest time of her life. They lived in a house of their own and were married for many years with their four children. Iron Man loved his wife very much, she was his dear sweet heart, as a surprise he even bought a nice car for her to go anywhere she wanted, she didn't have to travel anymore. She gained his trust, every weekend Saturday and Sunday she used the car to go to the market and the grocery for food stuff and other items that was needed for the home. Then from Monday to Friday she would take the children to school and so on, while her husband was at work.

Now most of the time she would be a house wife since Iron Man did not want her to work at all, anything she wanted that money could buy it was his pleasure to make sure she got it. It seems that they were a happy family and things were going good but she got a bit to comfortable.

Soon she started going out by herself in the day, without her husband knowing anything. She would cook and clean the house and leave, but she would always come back in time, at the normal time to get the children or do a chore. This went on for a long time until someone who knew me very well said, it's none of his business but he saw Iron Man's wife in a certain part of the country, with the said car that she was driving. It was parked at the side of the road and in the front seat was a tall dark, strong man, he and the Iron Man's wife spoke for over an hour.

I said okay but I didn't say anything. Now even though it was my neighbour, my good friend, it was also not my business because woman and man issue when behind closed doors is another thing. When those two making love to each other with one little sweetness in bed. Then he would remember and say: "Well I tell you honey, you know what Bany tell me?"

"Not now we go talk later honey," she reply and rock his world.

Then when he tell her, she say, "What? Ah seeing a next man behind yuh back, never!"

This is exactly what does happen so I left it alone.

Now talk does spread real fast and it was so that Iron Man eventually heard it from someone else. One day on my way to work, when I was just about to open my shop he came and said to me, lock up shop let's go for drive. Now I was wondering why and for what reason, anyhow I played along even though I had an idea of what was going on I said nothing. We went to a bar, we both sat down and talked. From observation, most Trinidadian men who get Mr. Horn will find themselves in a bar or pub, they would even go to a whore house with dancer girls around, looking on and drinking their problems away. They try hard for it to leave them. We may even go behind a next woman fast to try and fill that void in our hearts, a replacement that never works because at the end of it all, you will still be in a lonely corner.

While sitting and drinking some alcohol in a bar, he bring up the talk about his wife cheating on him and that he did not know how long this was going on for. He said it didn't matter because he always loved his wife, he admitted that he loved that woman so much that he would do anything to make her happy.

"We have four children together, one boy, three beautiful girls, my family is important to me and I cannot allow my family to break up now after so many years of marriage. It's hard, so hard, I love my wife so much."

Poor me again, ended up in the middle of them, having to be making decisions on what to do, even though we were neighbours and good friends for years, how could I do such a thing?

"Look how long we know each other as neighbours," he insisted. "This is the reason why I come to you and trust you with my problem, I really can't go to someone else okay."

"You know I have to get personal and ask you private questions," I told him.

"Go ahead," he said. "Ask me anything ah just want my family together, I just want to be happy again."

Well, all the questions was put to him concerning his wife but yet he was still in doubt. They say love is blind and that might be a fact in real life because he went on to ask me a very foolish question.

"You feel she really have a next man?" He asked.

What a question! After all you just tell me that she's not sleeping with you anymore and you cannot touch her. Your own wife when the night comes you cannot touch her and this was going on for months.

"Oh come on, what proof you need again," I answered.

After all our talk I admonished him to stay separate from his wife. "It will be a hard thing to do but it will be for your own good and well being. For now, just leave the thing as it is for the sake of the children. They may not understand the situation but once mummy and daddy together in the same house they good."

So things almost went back the same, but in a pretend state, it was not good two months after that meh girl belly started showing up. Now this even gave him more reason to put her out of their house because he said they not sleeping in the same bed, not having any kind of sex so he couldn't get his wife pregnant. So it was the hornerman child, so he did just that.

"You getting smart," I said to him.

Things worked out with their separation, she went to live with the hornerman and Iron Man stayed with his children. He took my simple advice and focused on his children.

There are consequences for horning, sometimes it may not be right away but down the road you will reap the benefits of this

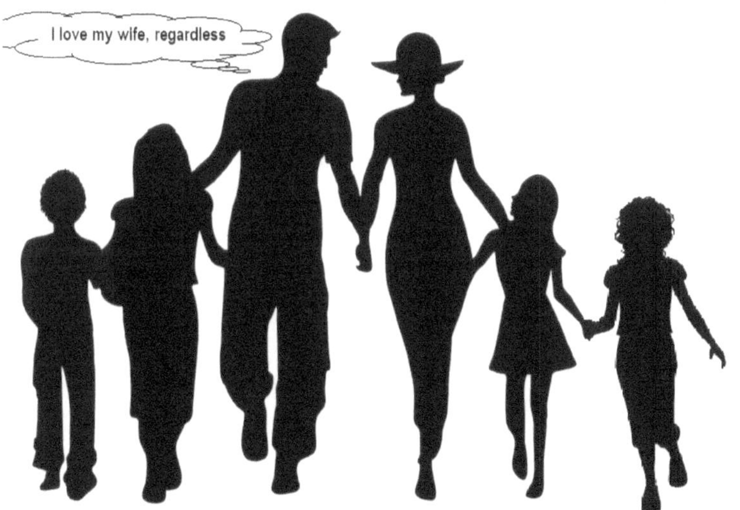

so-called love and temporal hour of pleasure. After living with the hornerman for a few years he became very Ill and was hospitalized, only to find out that he was in the stage of full blown AIDS. Doctors tried to treat and save him but they couldn't do anything for him at that stage. He spent a while in the hospital and eventually passed on.

My neighbours wife knowing what was taking place with her new man became frantic, this played with her mind. She took an overdose of pills and was going out of her mind. She took a bible and went to the streets and started preaching the word of God to people who passed in her transparent nightgown, you could see her underwear plainly. She created quite a stir on the streets and the police moved in and took her to a mental institution for tests.

I really don't know if while she was pregnant with the child if she ever visited a clinic or if she was tested for HIV, however the baby was born and always had health issues. She took treatment for a few years before dying with HIV/AIDS.

Up to this present day my neighbour would say, "Boy if it wasn't for you, I may not have been alive today."

"I tell him to give God thanks and praise." **"**

Chris and Baggy
The Classic Horn Story

" If you can't take horn then don't give horn.

Trouble easy to come but it's hard to go away. I was a victim of horn once, and I have experience in giving the horn as well. I've been there and done that but I tried to settle myself down and have a good life but when people don't want that, is horn all over again, until ah didn't even know myself, ah cyah sleep, nah eating, meh mind space out, ah feeling like a fool, sometimes ah want to dead, is all kind ah thing does take you.

When I feel what being horn feel like, it's really is, do so doh like so. It's a true saying that cheating can cost you your life, it can separate your good family members forever and make best friends turn enemies. You can get infected with HIV/AIDS, it can bring you shame among your friends and co-workers and what about your children? What example are you showing them, are they to do the same thing as you did? Is this what we call change in society? While the nation's children look at us as adults, is just big people getting on like children.

I am being real here, if I can write and share other people's stories, then I can also write about myself. It's only fair that I share about me, Chris and Baggy plus the hidden man to whom I thought she had done with.

In this story, basically there were three men who shared everything with one woman, thinking about it I never knew if I was placed first or even second much less for third. To be honest as a man you never know where you stand with women.

This girl Chris was living with a man already, but she wasn't married just common law/boyfriend-girlfriend thing. I can't remember every detail of how we met but as I go along I will write what I remember.

Chris started visiting me at the shop where I worked, this was years ago when I was a much younger man. We would talk for very long hours, conversations on almost any topic that came to mind, this turned out to be an interesting situation between the both of us, while speaking she would model around the floor with her hands on her hips swaying from left to right and watching me with a sexy smile. Her eyes were fixed in a seductive way, my eyes were also in a fixed position looking right back at her but blushing.

As a man at that moment my mind went blank, forgetting that she was already living with a man but she wasn't married which meant to me that she could leave him and come with me.

"Damn she looking good from head to foot," I drooled.
I snapped out of it and we exchanged numbers. About a week

after she called my phone for the first time and said we have to go up by mammy to fix an appliance. In those days I was a real good fix-it-appliance man alright, the best.

"Pick a day and time and give me directions as to where to meet you," I said.

We made arrangements to meet on a Friday afternoon, we meet and travelled up to her mother's place. Upon reaching there she introduced me to the family who were there at the time, then took me to the room that the appliance was located.

I looked through it and had it working in no time so Mammy asking Chris about me.

"Who is this one, is he your new boyfriend?" She asked openly.

"No, he is just the fix-it-man," Chris replied.
"Okay, so where is your shop located?" Mammy probed.

"Oh somewhere in this land," I joked.

Now Mammy seeing me as the new man, then this have me wondering how much man this girl really have or is seeing at a time.

Anyway, back in those days there were some jobs for me down the islands, it depended on the type of work that was needed to be done so it sometimes took two weeks to be completed. When that happened I needed workers, so I asked Chris, "Would you be able to join the crew and go down the islands to work with us?"

Now in my head, my intentions may have been good and bad at

the same time.

She agreed but still told me to ask her mother who was not standing far from us, and she would go for sure.

"Girl you crazy," I replied, "How could I do such a thing and you living with a man?"
She just smiled, so I went boldly to mammy and asked her.

"Go girl," mammy answered, "because that man you have can't give you nottin, so go and if he come here, I go deal with him."

When I hear that so, I could not like a better sport.

Then I asked foolishly: "Why don't you tell your boy-friend that you are going down the islands to work for about two weeks and you will be back with him very soon."

I knew very well that it would only be the both of us soon and was just being pretentious.
"No, ah ain't telling him nothing," Chris declared. "He will never let me go with any man, is only up by Mammy ah could go and besides he doh give me nottin. Is my mother does give me any-thing that I need."

With both of them standing in front of me, mother and daugh-ter I said, "Right now, I really didn't need any trouble with an-ybody."

"Mister this is my child and if ah tell she go, then go," Mammy said firmly.

"Okay mom," I agreed with a smile on my face.

We organized and bought up all that was needed to take on the boat and we were on our journey down the islands. It was Saturday evening about half past two, it took thirty minutes to reach. There were five separate houses on the island, each and every one packed away their stuff. While they were doing that Chris and I went for a walk around the small island space where people would fish at night.

We both sat on the rocks with our feet down in the water talking to each other, between our conversation she would bring up talk about this man her secret man, saying how he does treat her and that things not really good with them, so she's just there and all he does want is one thing.

"What is the one thing?" I ask.

She said what else more than sex.

"Girl," I said. "Hear what, we did not come here to talk about your hidden man, is not my business so keep that to yuh self, you come here to work and that's all."

I was really mad at that time. Then suddenly she stood up from behind the rock where we were sitting. Next thing you know is top coming off, then skirt sliding down. I was now only seeing white panties and bra, I was seeing heaven and then I saw hell but remain on earth still and motionless.

"What are you doing?" I asked.

She told me that she was taking a dip in the salt and wanted me to join her. What else could I do, I jumped into the water with all my clothes on. That was foolish of me because while we were in the water there was bouncing and touching, all kind of thing but no sex. We just played around having fun. Not too long after the beautiful sun set went down on the horizon and darkness began to fall into place, so it was time to go inside. The owner of the island asked us which house each one of us would be staying in.

"The last one to the top would do me fine," I replied.

Chris and the owner's wife were the only women on the island with us so I asked for her to sleep in a separate house from the others. We each went to our respective houses for the night, I locked up tight and sat looking through the window. Now it was very dark and cold on that island at night, but when you get a glance at the other islands with those yachts on the water, it was a beautiful sight. All the lights reflecting upon the dark water, roaring waves dashing against the rocks; seeing the white of the water diminish. I watched this for a while before going to sleep. The night was so cold that I wrapped myself around in a blanket and fell asleep quickly.

It was nearly midnight when I heard knocking on my door. Who could be knocking at the door at this hour? I wondered. I got up but didn't open it but the knocking continued.

"Who is it and why are you knocking at this hour?" I asked. Chris answered.

"What are you doing out there?" I asked as I opened the door. "What you want?"

"Boy," she said. "Ah cyah sleep, I not accustom being by myself so."

"What now?" I asked a bit confused.

"Boy ah want to sleep in the same house with you," Chris explained.

"Okay," I agreed. "You take the bed and I will sleep on the couch." So we both did just that and I went back to sleep. It was not long afterwards that I felt something coming up my cover by my feet and I jumped.

"What are you doing in there?" I asked quickly.

"Boy, I can't sleep still?" Chris explained.

"So what now?" I asked again.

"Just hug me up and I will fall asleep?" She declared.

Now this was not an easy thing to do, it was not possible for me to fall asleep so easy with this girl in my arms but I went along with it. As we lay there on the couch hugging, is one leg over my body and I asked: "What are you doing to me?"

"Do you like what yuh feeling?" She purred.

Well I am just human, of course I like what I was feeling.

"Do you want to feel more of me?" She continued.

Believe me when I say I reach a point of no resistance with Chris, I could not say no or refuse her. We caressed and kissed, we did not stop until the next morning. Afterwards I thought that I made a big mistake.

The next day we started to work on the project, depending on the workload sometimes we finished earlier than other days.

When all work was finished for the day we would go for a swim close to the shore around the island. Some parts were deep, other parts shallow. We had lots of fun, we even found ourselves doing wrong things in the water and each night we slept together.

The job was completed in one and a half weeks and we headed back to land. On the way home each person was transported to their destination until it was only Chris and I left to go home. The driver asked me where to so I told him we are dropping this girl home.

"No," she said, "ah going by Mammy, and not that man."

How it looking like for me, she don't want to go back by that man, here comes trouble. There is a song that goes like this: Think I'm in trouble, I should have run on the double.

"Girl where are you going?" I asked to make sure.

"Up by my mother," Chris insisted.

"What about your boy-friend?" I asked.

"I done with he," Chris answered.

"Why now?" I asked not feeling so brave.
"Because you are more fun to be around than him," she declared.

Problems started when de man looking all over for this girl. Even up by her mother she would be hiding while Mammy lying and saying Chris not here, ah doh know whey she gone.

At night I find myself going up by Chris liming very late, while her family watching TV is me and she loving up on the back step of the house. Sometimes on the neighbour wall with bright light shinning down on us. This went on for one year and then she decided to move in with me in my apartment. There were four houses in that yard, one house was for the land-lord and his son Baggy, the other houses were for his daughter and grand children. It was a very big yard. We live together for more than seven months there.

One day I noticed that Chris was not with me in bed when I got up. This happened for a while, after investigating I realized that she used to be liming with Baggy, sitting on the front steps of his door.

So I asked her what you doing there?

"Boy ah does come to make phone call," she answered.

I reminded her that we had two phone with money on it and wanted to know what nonsense was going on. From that day on I watching her reaction, there was something in the making there. Nevertheless she came back across into our apartment and stopped going by Baggy six o'clock in the morning.

Things continued good for a short while. Now there was a Saturday that she told me she was going by Mammy and I said no problem. I will go lime with my friend in the bar which was not too far from where we lived. I returned home about 1:30 a.m. that Sunday morning from liming with friends because she told me that she would be by mammy. It was a very warm night, so I opened my door and then headed to the stand pipe on the outside to have a bath because I couldn't sleep good without taking a bath. I heard a squeaking sound and stopped. I did not know where it was coming from so I stood still and listened to hear if I would hear it again and then it began to squeak like someone was ironing clothes to go out. So I wondered why would someone be ironing at half past one in the morning. I followed the squeaking sound which was coming from the back of the house. On reaching around the house I saw a man holding on to a woman bending her over in a position, while holding on to her two hands behind her back on an ironing board but I couldn't see clearly because the glass on the window was frosted. So I was seeing shadows and outlines but I kept on watching and saying to myself. Action yes! oh my gosh, ha!

Next thing the squeaking became louder, I stood there and kept saying action, then there were shouting. "Oh God Baggy! No Baggy! Stop Baggy! Baggy No, No, Baggy, No, No Baggy! Baggy! Baggy!

That is when I checked myself, only to realize that the voice sounding like my girl. Yes, it was at that moment that I tried to remain calm but I could not. I went into my apartment took up a three line cutlass in my hand and run up to that window to chop that glass away in rage, so I could see clearly what was taking place.

Then I dropped the blade, there were some rocks on the ground, I picked them up in both hands and charged. I was hoping to smash the window, I just wanted to see with my own eyes clear as it could be if this was really happening. Then I dropped the rocks. I finally took a piece of 2x4 wood in my hand and ran towards the window again. Then I dropped the wood.

What the ass was going on with me?

It was a historical moment in my life, then I calmed myself down and went to the front of Baggy door step and knock on it so hard, that my hand almost went through the door. Both of

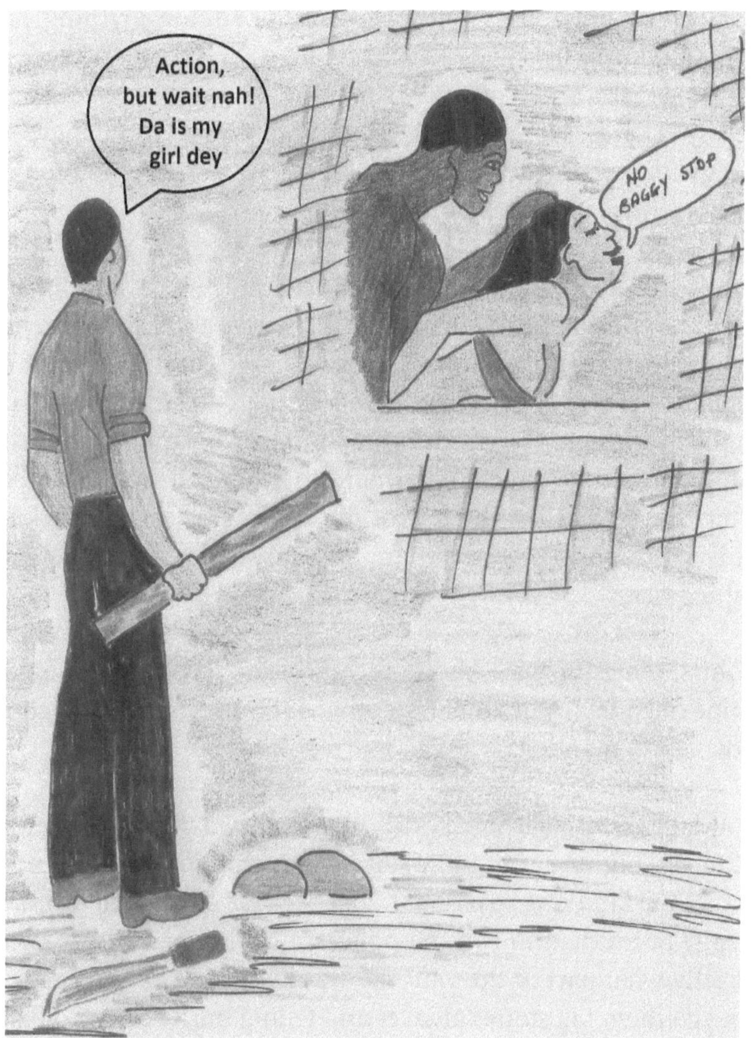

them quickly fighting up trying to put on clothes and open the door right after. She seeing me after one in the morning have the belly to ask me what I doing there?

Then I asked her the same question: "What are you doing here in Baggy house?"

"Oh we was not doing anything, we was not doing anything, just hanging out," Chris lied.

"Okay," I said. "How does this sound then. "Oh God Baggy, No Baggy, Baggy, Baggy! Girl I am sure it was not my name you calling. This is where Mammy is eh."

I took all my clothes that hour of the morning, went out the road, stopped a car, the driver ask me where and I told him just drive. He drove down town, then back up to the main for hours then dropped me off and I walked around town until about 5am in the morning. Afterwards I went home by my mother, but still had some things in the apartment to collect. It was one week after that I went for the rest of my stuff, while inside packing only to hear this girl first man, the one she say she done with calling her.

"Chris! Chris! Chris! Ah know yuh inside dey and you better come outside now if you know what good for you. You go come now," he demanded.

You talk about bacchanal. This man had two pigtail bucket fill of plenty big stones in it, he started launching/pelting them towards the landlord apartment. Just because of this one woman, Baggy father had to call the police since the man didn't know exactly what part of the yard she was living. So, he was just letting go them big stones all over and telling me he come to fight.

I said to him, me not fighting and killing myself over any woman. To calm things down I carry out her suitcase with clothes and give it to him saying. "Look yuh girl inside by Baggy, is he have yuh girl not me. You could take she and go."

"We never done," he said to me. "She just walk out on me."

The thing was she was done with him but he was never done with her.

This girl was a trap, I could not give all the details, this is what and how I remembered it. Up to this day each time I think of that situation I would laugh but before I could not laugh though.

This goes to show that when you see people in a relationship even if they are not going good, just listen please, don't get involved, stay away from these types of situations.

This could have ended in death, I could have even got sick with HIV/AIDS or any other killer disease. It could have been a big stone to my head or any other part of my body.

She was a games player, where three men came into a love triangle. It was from me, to Baggy, back to the other man, he even went on to say that Chris used to go back at night to have sex with him and neither me nor Baggy knew of this.

I always wondered, what if Baggy or the other man had HIV?

It all boils down to this even though one man could make love better than another man, at the end she was still going back to the same man, she was just bad. It made no sense at all, especially where your life is concerned.

I took a chance, like many of the others in these stories and that chance could have cost me my life. Sometimes this is part of life and a learning experience to know don't go there again because if you can't learn now, you will never learn again.**"**

Drinking Risk and Behaviour

"Going out on dates with friends can be a very risky situation when drinking in groups around tables with open glasses. Sometimes leaving and go to the washroom while your drink is still on the table is risky, someone may put a drop of Spanish Fly Pro in your drink and you will never know the difference because it blends in with the wine or whatever kind of alcohol you may have. After liming particularly if you are a single woman, men would take the opportunity to offer you a ride home hoping that the Spanish Fly Pro works on the way. Once this happens it makes you feel for sex immediately and since he will be the only man there he will oblige. This product makes you vulnerable, with all the alcohol together with Spanish Fly Pro in your head you won't even think of using a condom. This is where the risk of unprotected sex will begin.

I knew a French creole man in his late 70's, he taught me all about this product. Please don't get me wrong, I never tried this product on any one before or after learning about it. He went on to say to me that in his younger days he had many women friends and he would walk with a bottle of alcohol and Spanish Fly with each one who would invite him out and put it in her drink.

While cheers were taking place and glasses knocking together, if women only went to the wash-room for a few minutes, he said to me he would put enough Spanish fly in her drink, which he thought was the fastest way to get sex from that woman. He did this a few years well and today he has twenty-three children with several women all over the place. Now back then it was just Spanish-fly and it was effective if used properly but today it is a more advanced formula, more effective in use. This Spanish Fly Pro is a product that was made for women who had dif-

---

HOW TO USE NEW SPANISH FLY – SPANISH FLY PRO
https: www.spanishflypro.com/how-to-use/

The dosage of Spanish Fly Pro is pretty simple. All you have to do is mix 5-7 drops with any drink. It works best with any alcohol drink, such as wine and so on. Then, just wait for several minutes and prepare for the best sex of your life!

1. Put a few drops of Spanish Fly Pro into a beverage. 5 drops should be enough for every one but test it to find your personal dosage. Do not worry about over dosing as this is never an issue.

2. Mix it and Drink it: It works best with Red Wine or any other alcoholic drink. Do not combine with coffee or any other hot beverage. Wait a few minutes for the drops to take effect. 10 minutes should be enough. You can still help with setting the right mood and atmosphere.

Five drops of the product is all it takes to enjoy the bliss of sexual intimacy. If you use more the effect will be stronger, every girl needs a slightly different amount to get aroused. The amazing trait of the new and improved Spanish Fly pro is the speed at which it takes effect, after five minutes of taking the product a woman can already feel the stirring effects and promise of sexual pleasure.

It is clinically tested and worldwide approved. Spanish Fly Pro meets all of the requirements set out by the Federal Drug Administration of the USA. This means that this product is totally safe and sanctioned by recognized international regulating agencies. During a test conducted on 2600 couples for two months, 93.3% of the couples stated that their female partners noticed an increase in their sexual appetites and 84.2% of the female participants stated that sexual intercourse actually became more pleasant and they had multiple orgasms. An amazing feat indeed and all thanks to the Spanish Fly Pro which is now available on the market. The test further revealed that there was no negative side effects except when taken on over-dose. The negative side effect was very minimal though, with a very slight drowsiness all that was noted. Nothing else, just extreme sexual desire!

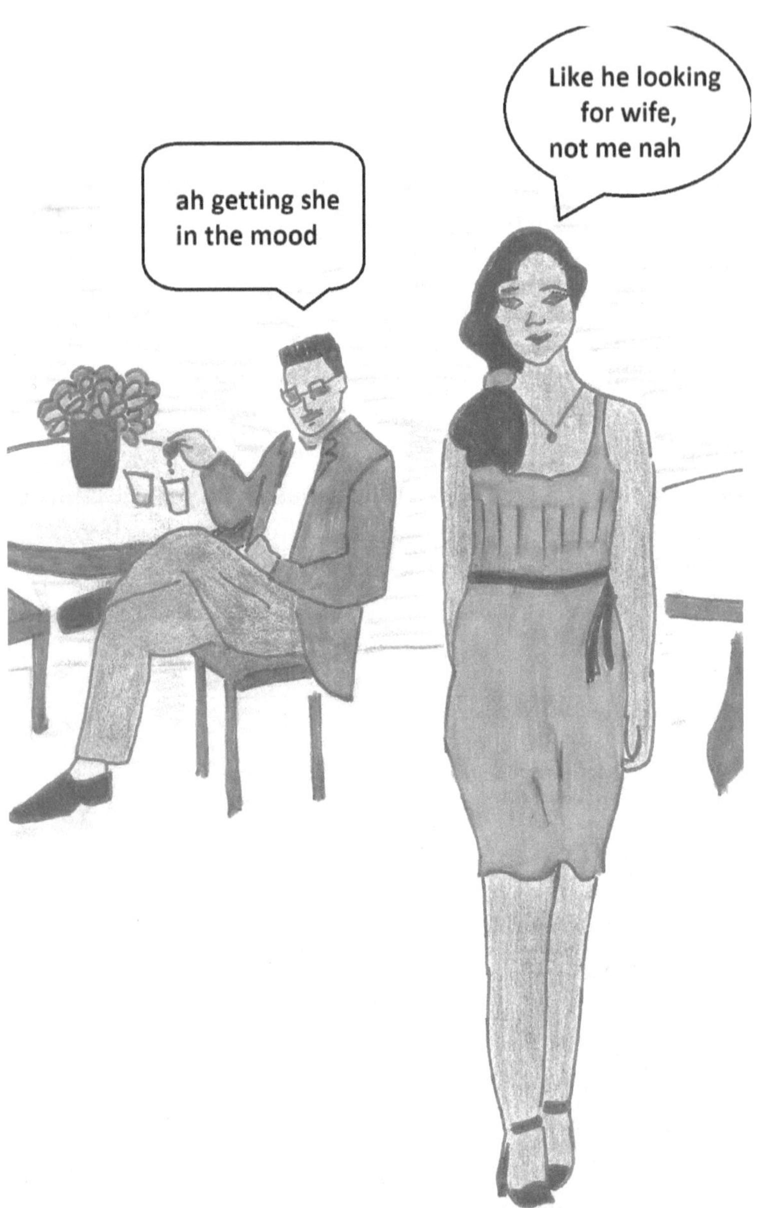

ficulties in reaching an orgasm. This is a quick way to stir up sexual desires with your partner but people today who are now learning about this brand are using it for all the wrong reasons and purposes. They are misusing it to their advantage and your disadvantage.

In our society some of our women on a whole just don't give a damn about who is around and who is watching them. The dress code of the day has no moral sense and standard, whatever we feel to put on, it's okay. It's fine to have on a two piece in your house but to then walk down town in broad daylight.

Who cares about people looking they say? What if my clothes run up my legs and every 10 second I have to pull it down?

"All I know is that ah looking good and dem man and dem does break dey neck watching me pass because I have wha it takes to turn heads."

I guess this is the style going. Many many years ago I walk into a police station to make a report, upon reaching the front desk one of the police officers said to me. "Come forward and make your report."

Just when I was about to do so, everything in the front portion of the police station come to a halt. Only to see standing close by a browned skinned, slim, nice, beautiful, young, sexy lady who also came to make a report. This was the most ridiculous moment standing there watching all those police officers forget everyone else and focus on this one individual. They allowed her to make a report, only to realize that I had been put on hold because all of their attention was on this young woman.

Now all this was the report she made, while standing there listening she said: "Officer I was walking down the road and this fella see me and started harassing meh but I continued to go about my business officer. He kept on after me, when I see him coming, fright come upon me and I began to run but he was also running fast towards me. Nobody was there, he grabbed me from behind holding on to my hair. I tried to scream but he pointed a knife at me and place his hands over my mouth. He was much stronger than me, he laid me down on the ground, ripped my shorts pants off of me and raped me, over and over repeatedly until he satisfied himself. He was all smiling while I was in tears trying to pull myself together. He then ran into some nearby bushes. Officer I felt sick, sick.

After those officers heard the story one of the officers come out from behind the desk and walk towards the girl looking at her steady saying: "Look, what you had on eh! Look what you wearing. Watch the short pants you have on and all your belly outside this is how you come out the road eh. You must want to get rape because you exposing everything. What you expect eh?"

Now this incident here is an example of what other women went through at similar conditions, even though she may put up a fight with the individual, she was no match with him due to his strength and weapon of choice that was being pointed right at her, which I think would make her physically handicap.

I clearly remembered in this other story where I once lived in a village, there were just a few of us coming together in a house to keep a prayer meeting on Tuesday and Thursday night. What I noticed that the others didn't, was a single girl who would arrive late each and every session.

She would appear almost when the meeting was nearly finished and I wondered why was that because she wasn't living that far. Upon suspecting and investigating, I realized to my surprise that she left home a little bit before the prayer meeting would start, she would leave home and stop by a man and talk for long hours outside his gate.

This went on for a while then she started going inside by this man with the doors closed for the long hours then she came to the prayer meeting all sweaty and smelling weird. Everyone would wonder why she was always coming so late but no one knew more than I.

This went on for almost a year it did not stop there, when I looked during the day time from Monday to Sunday this girl would wash and cook and put food and clothes in a bag, each and every day at a certain hour to carry for this man next door.

So I decided to ask a question. "Why are you washing and cooking for this man and spending hours when you go into his room?" I asked her one day. "Is this your boy-friend?"

She said no.

"Are you in a relationship with him?" I asked.

She said no.

"Do you know that he is a bandit?" I asked.

She told me yes, that she was aware of that. She was doing this out of fear. She said the man showed her a gun and told her if she didn't cook and wash and give him sex when he wanted then he would shoot her.

"Did you use a condom?" I asked her.

No, she replied.

"He does like it just so," she admitted. She went on to say that she was on birth control pills.

The man also told her that if she told anyone he would shoot her.

"Now brother for Christ sake don't tell anybody," she begged, "because ah feel he go kill meh. Please don't tell anyone about this."

Now did you see the picture here, he did not point a gun at her head and rape her but just the idea that he showed the gun to her, and with his powerful words of fear and threats, which he injected into her mind, he made this girl do things by force that she never intended to do.

So you see in the first story the woman who made the report got raped the same instance but that was once but in the other story my friend was raped technically for almost a year by this man through fear, even though she didn't want to or feel like it, she gave in.

For me both of these situations was rape, it was just different situations.

This remained between the young lady and myself until today, no report was ever made to the police station, not even her mother and family knew. However she gained VISA entry into the USA and is currently living a new life. In the meanwhile the bandit who was responsible for these actions against this girl was shot by police just a few years after. He is now walking with a stick in order to balance his body. **"**

Rape Victim

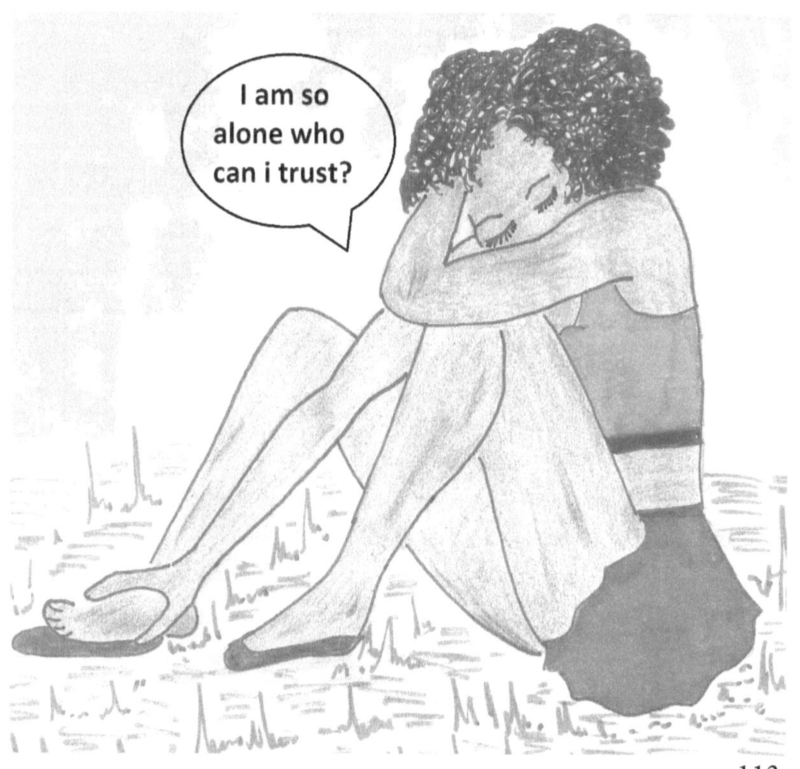

"There are situations where a woman can become a vulnerable and helpless victim of rape and sexual abuse. Being raped at gun point or even knife point or any other weapon is just as dangerous and risky. This may not give a woman much choice but to cooperate with the stranger either you are wounded or killed.

In these instances whether it is a single man or a group of men, we all know that a raper-man don't have time to put on condoms. They do not care that you are HIV positive, they may be sick with that or other diseases but the idea is only one thing they are seeing and that is all their focus is on. Remember this is not his property or belongings, it is an illegal act of thieving sex from another man's wife, or someone's sister or even a mother's daughter.

These type of acts are considered to be force upon by invading one's privacy with painful penetration into the vagina giving sex without your consent or permission.

This way is a quick act of aggressiveness and the urge to discharge as fast as possible into their victim by satisfying their own lustful ways. It matters not how you feel or think, it's all about them, now the after effects brings more questions than answers:

1. What if I have contracted HIV?

2. What if I am pregnant?

3. How will I live with myself?

4. Maybe all men are the same?

5. Should I report this to the police?

6. If I report it, will my life be in danger?
7. Can I tell my best friend?

8. What about the man who rape me, he was known to me for many years so now what?

9. Should I keep this to myself?

10. What if he tells other people?

11. They may say I wanted it for a long time. Am I the one who asked for it?
12. I don't think I want a next man ever again. What should I do about a situation like this?

This will now leave me scarred, traumatized, mentally disturbed and physically challenged with scars for the rest of my life. Sometimes good counselling and talking to a close friend will help, it takes time to heal.

Life is strange people who we put our trust in are sometimes the ones that do us harm while the people we do not trust are the one's who will comfort us. **"**

Living Common Law

"When trini couples live common law or marry there are situations or problems that will arise out of a simple matter where you need to be a big person, you can sit and talk about it but instead one may start a quarrel that may go like this.

Situation 1

"Girl look how long we together babes ah not throwing back nothing in yuh face but all them things I do fuh yuh over the years eh, I furnish de house, and even put you in it. What about the car I bought you eh?"

"Look boy watch nah, all them furniture you talking about is old thing that was more than twenty years old since in your grandmother days and you see that old car you give meh dey, it always breaking down all over the place. Only embarrassment is man does have to stop and help me push it just for it to start up. Boy what you ever give me? What you ever do for me? You never give me nottin a real man doh talk about something he already give to a woman eh. Is vex you vex why you bringing up all them things nah."

"Girl change yuh ways for once nah, oh gosh. Is best you go from here yes."

"Well if that is the case ah leaving, ah going with everything in the house."

"Girl you mad so you ain't leaving nothing for me?"

"Boy I work hard for that you know!"

"How?"

"All them positions, cleaning this house, cooking food for yuh, washing clothes for you and yuh mother like a slave and plenty of love whenever you need it."

"So then our love never count, it doh mean a thing? You sounding like the ole hoe[19] or some kinda hustler."

19 A whore

"Boy hall yuh ass nah, look boy doh get me on the wrong side this morning you hear! I fed up of you. You just like a woman always quarrelling. Is best you was wearing panty and bra, you would ah get a good fit and all them man would run you down. Take what I telling you, is best yuh was a woman, yuh mother make the wrong child."

"Girl hush up now nah, ah tired of hearing you, ah does cyah take that mouth you have dey, give it a rest, oh gosh man so everybody have to hear we business an wha going on in dey house?"

"Well hush meh up nah, do meh something nah boy."

"Girl if I follow you police will take meh, ah go make a jail."

"You mean is the other way around, you ain't see my size to you? All I have to do is sit down on you and put one leg across yuh skinny ass and all fight done. So if you know what good for yuh, you go behave yourself."

"Come nah babes leh meh give you a hug."

"Man doh touch meh, man move nah, leh meh go. You feel you could tell meh all them hurtful things and then talk back to me. It doh work so yuh know."

"Girl what ah go do without you in my life, you are meh wife, meh everything. If you leave me now ah feel ah go dead."

"Well dead."
"I reach a stage babes that I can't live without you in my life, so ah sorry. Please forgive meh."

"Okay ah forgive yuh but for the next two months I want you to do all the house work and every night you are going to massage my back for me, plus bring me breakfast in bed."

"Yes honey, anything for you."

"You sure?"

"Yes love."

"Also I am putting you on probation."

"What kind of probation?"

"No sex of any kind until I say so."

"But girl you mad, you crazy. How you could do that to me?"

"Is alright I go see what could work out."

"Now that sounding much better love. Okay ah hungry after all that quarrelling go cook something for we honey."

"Ah going."

Situation 2

"Look at him going dey, like them panty man and them, damn fool if you know how I vex with myself now, ah should of listen to my mother, ah feel ah make a mistake marrying this blasted man. What ah give him to eat like it rub off on meh life. Wha ah go do, just go with the flow and see how things work out for both of us after God.

Situation 3

"You see me, I fed up, he and me done because everything I do is a problem. They say the devil find work for idle hands, something just come to meh mind. Ah better try a ting and see. I wonder whey meh phone is? Yes look right here leh me call Paul and see what he doing now."

Ring, ring, ring ...

"Paul, yes meh husband just leave."

"How you know that the man was cooking and he done so he went out the road."

"Ah really don know where he gone but ah doh business so what you for?"

"Well girl I for anything right about now."

"Paul what to do, come across by you or you will come over."

"Girl I doh want to take a chance, is best you come over by me instead, okay."

"On my way."

Knock, knock, knock ...

"Well Paul open the door nah, do fast, ah not supposed to be seen coming in here."

"Come girl, come fast. Oh my, ooh my gosh babe, you looking real good and nice from ever since, big bottom, small waist hah, ah tell yuh, you know how long ah want you."

"Boy stop touching meh an feeling meh up, what happen is hurry yuh hurry so? You getting on like you thirsty, you can't wait?"

"Well then why you come here girl?"

"Alright nah, you have condoms though?"

"Ah going and look, ah nothing there, let me check in the cabinet here. I still searching."

"Look what happen so long you looking and you can't get not even one condom."

"Girl ah not seeing none!"

"So how we doing this thing now eh, you tell me?"

"Well ah go jump off fast, fast."

"Boy you know them kind of stunt doh work right and that is a chance I taking because two things can happen here, I could get pregnant and also HIV infected."

"Oh gosh girl how you could say them thing, I clean, yuh fully well know you safe with me."

"Boy ah not trusting nobody but God and you know ah living with ah man. Like you want me dead. Paul hear what, I doh know but with you, no condom no sex."

"But girl you waste my time eh, done get me in a mood."

"It's not you alone in that mood but at the same time I not risking my life for the sake of pleasing you because my whole future is ahead of me."

"Girl come nah, look how yuh have meh begging, is only once yuh giving me it, not twice eh. Look how long I waiting for dis day. Just give me a chance nah girl?"
"Boy stop begging, no is no you hear. What you just say? Once and ah chance, ah go take. Paul whey you feel I is them clothes pin gyal and them when you squeeze their head they legs does open eh? Ah pass them stage already. Ah girl could get sex any time, any where, you understand."

"Yes babe."

"Doh call meh dat."

Situation 4

Hear nah, a friend and I had a good conversation, this person literally beg me to try my best because at times we find ourselves compromising with a new boy-friend or girl-friend, on the use of condoms.

If you don't have condoms in the heat of the moment what will you do?

Which one of the members on your body will you control the most?

Is it to control your lower member or the upper one?

Some of us want to have two brains at the same time, which makes you indecisive. Why you go take a chance, and if you did why scratch your head after?

The truth here will be revealed since I take ah chance.

Now this is my story.
"With sniffling runny nose, it's like a flu symptom, that runs down my lips and never drys.

With a shrinking looking face, sucking inwards, now you can see the visibility of my cheekbones.

With so little hair left on my head, it's forever falling off, now I am bald.

With my stomach bubbling three to four times a day, only bowel movements back and forth in the washroom.

With these sores, look at the sores bursting out from my head to my feet.

With a grievous itchy rash on my neck, back, chest. It's even on my tongue and private area.

With my insides feeling hot and burnt up all the time, is real pain night and day, I am so restless.

With irregular fever, it comes and goes. My body is shivering now, uncontrollable shaking from sunrise to sunset.

With a lean type skeleton frame, my body is too weak to find it's balance when I walk.

With my body odor, it changes to a different type of unusual decaying smell.

With numerous complaints and complications, I know there is a fight against time between my red blood cells and the white ones.

With this HIV, it's AIDS now.

With tremendous weariness, in antagonizing frustration which now leave me with the stigma.

They calling me names, people talking to you but still distancing themselves. I see them, no one wants to sit in the same seat as I did a   second ago.

No one wants to drink in the same cup with you, no one wants to hug you much less shake your hand.

They watch me with scorn and sometimes pity, thinking they not coming close to me. They saying is better me than them yes.

With tears in my eyes I would cry over and over again until I fall asleep, knowing damn well if I ever wake up this is what I have to face over again.

It's a fight that I never give up or give into and people don't understand because this death is one of fear.

Yes, there is hope and people can live a normal, healthy life style with treatment but there is also this life, the one of pain and slow death that is always looming.

Always pray to God above." **"**

What is love?

"Girl, whole day ah calling yuh phone and yuh not answering."

"Well ah was by mammy helping she wash clothes in the machine so I couldn't hear meh phone ringing, okay nah, forget that."

"Come honey, I need to ask yuh something."

"What?"

"Yuh love meh?"

"Boy, you always asking me that, if ah doh love yuh ah wouldn't be here with you. Boy stop touching meh nah, look stop kissing me up and why you always biting me?

"What happen yuh doh like that?"

"No, because yuh does bite me hard, yuh is a dog or something. You know ah doh like too much ah dat!"

"Wait nah, wha is dat perfume smell ah getting here?"

"What smell you getting?"

"Girl like you have ah next man ah what? Like you horning meh?"

"But ah was by mammy whole day."

"Well call she nah. You little bitch, yuh hoe like you."

"Look who calling me hoe. Boy how much times when I ain't home you does bring woman right in de house to have sex with them eh and when I ready for you, yuh does cyah do nottin. You like them one minute man, ah should say 30 seconds and you done."

"Girl like is two ah we horning each other."

"Alyuh men does not know a good woman when yuh see one, you men does fuss about everything and always complaining that is why we woman does have alyuh men chupidee[20]. We does make all kinda songs just to make alyuh feel good, to make alyuh think yuh doing something and when everything done yuh telling all yuh padners and them next day, boy I cut she throat last night and ah have she crying out meh name; ah blaze she like that, ah give she good last night."

*****

"There is something I noticed every-time my girl go by she mammy, that bitch always coming back home with red spots on her neck and bottom. Boy like is all over she body and you know she done red skin and sexy. When ah ask she why she only coming back with red spots there, hear what she told me.

Boy is not no hickey, is mosquito that bite me dey and ah scratch it with my fingernails, that is why it looking so.

Like I foolish or something."

*****

"I know for a fact that there are lots of misunderstanding in re-lationships. There is a lost in communication and trust for each other and even a lack of respect for one another. This is some-thing that has been going on in our society, even around the world. For example some women would horn their man with a next man who don't give them anything.

---

20 *Stupid*

This weird tradition may be part of our culture, where she taking all your money and giving it to a hidden man who can't give her a thing in return more than just sex. This man not working anywhere but she's taking care of him, he comes and it's grab, slap, bend over sex."

"Boy ah love yuh," she professes.

"Girl move from here, go from here, what yuh telling me about love, is just fun we for," he responds.

"But I thought yuh love meh?" She goes on.

"Girl I could say anything now. Go meet yuh man," he laughs.

"So yuh doh want meh again?" She continues.

"Girl, we not together, yuh forget yuh man home? This was just a fling, a one night stand thing."

"... But my breasts much bigger and firmer, my legs are thick, my bottom is big and nice just how you like it. You like how I do it eh?"

"Girl, I doh need that from you again."

"Why now?"

"... Because ah badman have many girls, all kind and type ah boy could call on at any time so you see go from here, you have a man waiting on you bitch!"

"You is a dog you was only using me."

"Well I never rape you remember you give me it willingly. Babe doh cry nah, you know when ah want you ah would call you."

"You does always tell meh that and then fool meh."

"Oh gosh, doh cry, ah love yuh, doh cry."

*****

"These days it's not about love and the heart anymore it is all about money and material things. We are attracted to physical appearance: "Ah like them red, if yuh ain't red yuh dead; she lips pink it does make meh feel to kiss she up all day; I like how she does walk and wine[21]. I like them thick with plenty meat: ah like them slim and nice, small hips and waist; not too dark coco-brown jus right; ah like she shapely like God take he time with that bottom and make she."

Today in our society like you have to pick one, he loves me now then he loves me not: she loves me now then she loves my pocket. For me what I rather and prefer I don't know what I want best. I will take all of them.

Some say why marry and lock down them-self when they could live it up and have sex with no responsibility. It is only competition, as to who could do it better and last longer; who have bigger then smaller; no honey if you don't get the money; no money no love.

We are like foreign exchange transactions where we have to trade something for something."

---

21 *Moving your waist in a sultry or sexy motion when you walk or dance*

We Behaviour

"These are some of the behaviour of some trini-women who are involved with more than one sexual partner."

One : Glen
Characters: Glen, Mr. Jones, Rocky and Romeo

"Girl hear nah, you see Glen he does give meh when ah want it and how ah like it any day, any time and when yuh hear he done with meh so girl, ah does have to sit down side ways."

"Nah girl he is an animal or something?"

"Me ain't know but he good like that until ah does fall asleep fast - knock out cold till next day. My man home doh want nothing with Glen."

Two : Mr. Jones
"Well you see Mr. Jones he cyah do a ting to me, doh matter how ah try with that man."

"But ah find he does look so strong and healthy girl."

"That is only looks, you ain't know nah."

"... But how you could say ah thing like that?"

"Because he doh have nottin down dey, but you know ah love him bad because he money so nice and is so ah eating it out."

"What yuh go do with he?"

"I have a man who does give me it right up."

Three: Rocky

"Nobody could say nothing about Rocky?"

"Why girl?"

"This man is one of the best man I ever come across every month end before he go home to he wife, I is the first person he does pass by and girl half of he salary is mine. That is for meh nails, meh hair, meh toes, ah get pedicure, ah need clothes, gold chain and them thing, girl, he does show me real love and much care."

"… But no sex at all, at all so that man only for material things?"

"Well play yuh doh know is that nah."

Four: Romeo

"I think Romeo is one of a kind. No man never make me feel this way before he does make sure me and my son doh stay hungry. With him my house have everything in it and girl if ah want a KFC[22] ah getting that with a flick of a finger."

"Well girl if that man doing all them thing you must be does give it up right?"

"Girl wha yuh talking about, sex?"

"Yes, what else?"

"Yuh mad ah wha, he never see what that look like and he never will see it."

"Hear what nah you see behind close doors nobody could tell

---

22 *Popular Fried Chicken*

you, understand and stop lying on your vagina."
"Well sometimes, ah not lying if ah feel to give him a little thing in between you know ah go compromise that is to have him coming back because ah does need de money bad, bad."

"You can say what you want I working and not robbing no man, ah making ah living is something for something,"

"Doh mine meh business out here, it good to have a spare tyre."

Risk Behaviour of Persons

What causes people to get HIV/AIDS

https://www.healthlinkbc.ca/health-topics/HW151408

HIV infection is caused by the human immunodeficiency virus. You can get HIV from contact with infected blood, semen, or vaginal fluids. Most people get the virus by having unprotected sex with someone who has HIV. Another common way of getting it is by sharing drug needles with someone who is infected with HIV.

- Would rather use the word blood transfusion, it is the next most popular way in which people contract HIV. It may be possible to catch HIV through unprotected oral sex, but the risk is much lower, the risk is higher if the person giving oral sex has mouth ulcers, sores or bleeding gums.
- Having spontaneous sex, anytime, anywhere that you can jack up someone.
- Knowing someone well and trusting them enough to make you feel to have unprotected sex.
- Desperation, the urge that you need to have sex. I must have it because ah does get lots of headaches, I need a release.
- Drinking, getting drunk not knowing what is going on in your head, smoking a joint that makes you lose your head, being gay - having same sex partners - man with man and woman with women. In my opinion and experience flirting with someone by exchanging photos of your body or even phone sex and videos can lead to unprotected sex.
- Also persons who practice prostitution for money or drugs.
- Paying for sex or blow jobs.
- Sharing needles, syringes and other injecting equipment.
- From mother to baby before or during birth; by breast feeding
- For the HIV negative partners, receptive and anal. Sex (bottoming) is the highest risk sexual behavior but you can also get HIV from insertive anal sex (topping).
- Contact between broken skin, wounds or mucous membranes and HIV infected blood contaminated body fluids.

- Deep, open mouth kissing if both parties have sores or bleeding gums and the blood from HIV-positive partner gets into your blood stream. HIV is not spread through saliva.

Symptoms of HIV

How can you know if you have HIV?

During this period the immune system is learning to recognize HIV. The primary infection refers to the time when you are first infected with HIV. Within two to four weeks after infections, you may experience flu-like symptoms such as fatigue, fever sore throat, swollen lymph nodes, headache, loss of appetite or skin rash.

HIV is like a volcano in the crust of a planetary mass object such as the Earth, that allows hot lava, volcanic ash and gases to escape from a magma chamber below the surface waiting for erupting in the final stage.

Within a month or two of HIV entering your body 40% to 90% of people experience flu-like symptoms known as acute retro-viral syndrome (ARS) but sometimes HIV symptoms don't appear for years, sometimes even decades after the infection.

"In the early stages of infection the most common symptoms are none," says Michael Horberg PHD. Here are some of the symptoms that follows: fever; chronic fatigue; rapid weight loss; cough and shortness of breath; recurring fever; chills; night sweats; rashes; sores or lesions in the mouth, nose on genitals under the skin; sore throat; severe headaches; lymphoma; pneumonia; colon cancer; tuberculosis (TB); cytomegalo virus (Herpes); dehydration; depression; achy muscles; joint pain; swollen lymph nodes; peeling or cracking of lips; nausea; vomiting; persistent diarrhoea; nail changes; yeast infection; confusion or difficulty concentrating; tingling and weakness all over; menstrual irregularities.

All these lead to complications in the body and may or may not lead to a bad stroke. A stroke was recognized as an HIV complication since the early stages of the epidemic. Potential causes of stroke in HIV-1 includes opportunistic infections - tumours, atherosclerosis autoimmunity, cougulopathies, cardiovascular disease and direct HIV-1 infection of arterial wall.

Candidiasis is a common HIV related infection, it causes inflammation and a thick white coating on the mucous membranes, at your mouth, tongue, esophagus and vagina.

Cryptococcal Meningitis is an inflammation of the membranes and fluids surrounding your brain and spinal cord. This is a common central nervous system infection associated with HIV, caused by a fungus found in soil.

Toxoplama is a potentially deadly infection, it is caused by toxoplasma gondii, a parasite that spreads primarily by cats, infested cats pass the parasites in their stools and the parasites grows in your intestines and bile ducts leading to severe chronic diarrhoea in people with AIDS.

Tuberculous (TB) is the most opportunistic infection associated with HIV and is the leading cause of death among people living with the disease.

The Cytomegalo virus is a common herpes virus that is transmitted in bodily fluids such as saliva, blood, urine, semen and breast milk. A healthy immune system inactivates the virus and it remains dormant in your body, however if your immune system weakens, the virus re-surfaces causing damage to your eyes, digestive tract, lungs or other organs.

There are other symptoms that people can get swelling of glands around the neck and penis area, swelling lymph or glands under your arms, behind your ears, between your legs or private parts. This is the next stage of HIV.

Some of the people I knew told me that inside their body feels like a fire was burning up and I noticed that they drank a lot of cold water, malta[23] or smaltas to cool the heat down.

You cannot get HIV from

You can only get HIV from someone who is already infected with HIV through very specific ways, you cannot get it from:

- Touching someone who has HIV. The fact is HIV cannot survive outside of the body so you won't get HIV from touching someone, hugging them or shaking their hands. Sweat, exchanging food by hands, sleeping next to a person, drinking from the same cup or kissing them on the face.

- Using the same toilet seat, tables, door handles, cutlery or sharing towels. HIV doesn't survive on surfaces either, so you can't get HIV from any of these.

- The mere air. HIV cannot survive in the air so coughing or sneezing or spitting cannot transmit HIV.

- Water: The same applies here, HIV cannot survive in water, so you won't get HIV from swimming pools, baths, showers areas, washing clothes or drinking water.

- Food and cooking utensils. HIV cannot be passed on through food or cooking utensils, even if the person preparing your food is living with HIV.

- Tattoos and piercing. There is only a risk here if the needle used by the professional has been in the body of an HIV infected person and not sterilized afterwards. However most practitioners are required to use new needles for each client. I think barbering

23 *Popular Malt drink*

and salons should come under tools and machines sterilizing and changing of new blades for every client.

What happens when a person finds out that they are HIV positive?

Well few people can accept that this is the way it is, while others can. There are many persons living with HIV who take treatment after testing positive for HIV and there are those who are afraid to go for the test, this is an undisclosed number of persons.

No one likes the idea of having to live life with this sickness for the rest of their God given life. It is a nightmare that can kill you faster by thinking about it. Sometimes you may feel depressed and alone not wanting to eat or drink or having any one around you.

You are either HIV positive (infected) or HIV negative (not infected).

Is there a cure for HIV/AIDS

[https://www.sfaf.org/resource-library/hiv-faqs/]
There is no cure for HIV or AIDS meaning that there is no procedure or medication which has been scientifically proven to reliably eliminate the virus from a person's body or reverse the damage to the immune system.

There have been many advances in HIV treatments and therapies in recent years that have dramatically improved the quality of life for people with HIV. People are living longer and healthier with HIV than we used to think was possible.

There are also people whose bodies naturally suppress the virus without medication (referred to as "elite controllers"), though this happens rarely. Even some elite controllers opt to take anti-retro virals to reduce the damage caused by HIV to their immune system. One well studied but not yet replicated of a person who has been functionally cured of HIV is Timothy Brown, also known as "the Berlin Patient." You can read about the science behind the Berlin patients case online.

The term "functionally cured" means that the person doesn't have to take medications and there's so little of the virus in their body that they aren't being affected by it and can't infect anyone else. It's not 100 percent clear whether or not this will remain true in the long term. Other cases of HIV infected infants born to HIV or HIV positive mothers that were given anti-retro viral medications soon after birth that had been thought to be functionally cured of HIV. The "Mississippi Baby" maintained an undetectable viral load off of anti-retro virals for more than two years, but eventually the virus did return and began replicating.

A young French woman infected during birth and given early treatment is described as being in "remission" since she has maintained an undetectable viral load for 12 years off treatment. Other French adults, known as the VISCONTI cohort, who received early HIV treatment have maintained undetectable viral loads even without anti-retro viral therapy. It is not clear if these "post-treatment controllers" will suppress HIV replication in the long-term or if the virus will return as it did in the case of the Mississippi Baby.

Scientists validate lemon as possible cure for cancer, HIV

https://guardian.ng/features/health/scientists-validate-lemon-as-possible-cure-for-cancer-hiv/

In recent times there have been claims and counter claims on the use of lemon (Citrus limon) to effectively treat degenerative diseases such as cancer and Human Immuno-deficiency Virus (HIV)/ Acquired Immune Deficiency Syndrome (AIDS).

Results of a study published September 2017 in Journal of Advanc-

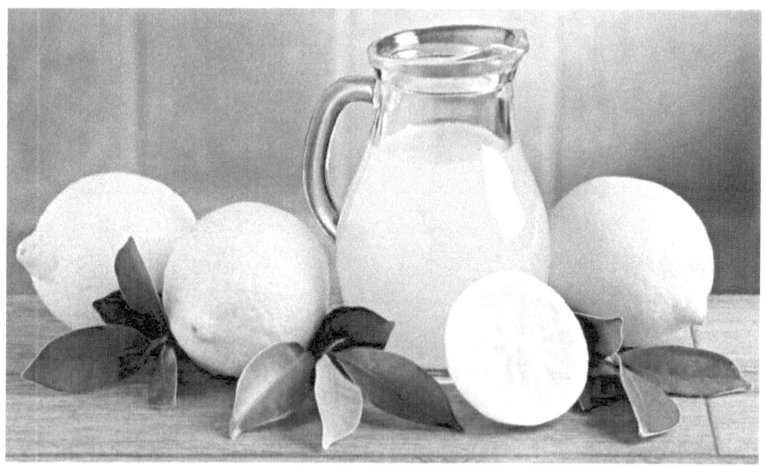

es in Molecular Biology suggest that lyophilized pure fruit juice powder of lemon has anti-proliferative effect against human breast cancer (MCF-7) cell line by suppressing its growth. The Indian researchers from Presidency College Chennai concluded: "Our results showed that lyophilized pure fruit juice powder of Citrus limon inhibited the proliferation of human breast cancer cell line MCF-7 with an IC50 98.16 µg/ml at 48 h incubation, it was shown to promote apoptosis as seen as Deoxy ribonucleic Acid (DNA)/ genetic material fragmentation using ladder assay. These results suggest that lyophilized pure fruit juice powder of Citrus limon has anti-proliferative effect against MCF-7 cell by suppressing its growth."

Excerpt below:

However, further experimental and clinical studies are needed to exploit the beneficial aspects of these juices and their extracts in full. The systematic review included and discussed twenty preclinical studies in which Citrus juices or their extracts were used as anticancer agents. In particular, twelve papers evaluated the effect of Citrus juices in in-vitro experimental models, and eight in in-vivo ones. Also, Australian researchers had reported that laboratory tests show that lemon juice is a potent destroyer of both HIV and sperm. The team at Melbourne University, led by Roger

Short, said if planned tests in primates and people are successful, lemon juice could be ideal for women without easy access to safe barrier contraceptives, such as condoms. But experts in anti-AIDS medications warn that the safety of using the juice internally and its efficacy in people are as yet unknown. Short said a solution of 10 per cent lemon juice produced a 1000-fold reduction in HIV activity in a lab sample. And half a teaspoon of the juice wiped out two teaspoons of sperm in 30 seconds.

The high acidity of the juice is responsible for killing HIV and sperm. Short said the great advantage of lemon or lime juice as an anti-viral contraceptive is that the fruit can be grown very cheaply in the developing world. He said women might use the juice by inserting a soaked piece of sponge or cotton wool before intercourse. Women researchers in Short's lab said using the juice caused no pain. Another study published in Phytomedicine validated the use of lemon juice and lemon grass (Cymbopogon citratus) for the treatment of oral candidiasis in an HIV population by the randomised controlled trial. They noted: The purpose of the study was to investigate the safety and efficacy of lemon juice and lemon grass (Cymbopogon citratus) in the treatment of oral thrush in HIV/AIDS patients when compared with the control group using gentian violet aqueous solution 0.5%. Oral thrush is a frequent complication of HIV infection. "In the Moretele Hospice, due to financial constraints, the treatment routinely given to patients with oral thrush is either lemon juice directly into the mouth or a lemon grass infusion made from lemon grass (Cymbopogon citratus) grown and dried at the hospice. These two remedies have been found to be very efficacious therefore are used extensively. Gentian violet, the first line medication for oral thrush in South Africa, is not preferred by the primary health clinic patients due to the visible purple stain, which leads them to being stigmatized as HIV-positive. Cymbopogon citratus and Citrus limon have known antifungal properties.

Citrus one of the important economically plants, but attention leaves and seeds the role of citrus not given importance in comparison to fruits despite the presence of phenols quantity that varies among species. Majority of citrus fruits are preferably eaten fresh example, oranges, mandarins, grapefruits, clementines, and tangerines. Orange and grapefruit produce very palatable juice and hence are used to make nutritious and popular breakfast.

Lemon is an important medicinal plant of the family Rutaceae. It is cultivated mainly for its alkaloids, which are having anti-cancer activities. Its fruits have peculiar fragrance partly due to flavonoids and limonoids present in the peel and these fruits are good sources of vitamin C and flavonoids. Lemons and limes can be used to make lemonades and pickles and their juices can be added to various food preparations as flavoring agents.

Citrus fruits are rich sources of active compounds and beneficial for human health example, vitamin C, carotenoids, flavonoids, limonoids, essential oils, acridone alkaloids, minerals, and vitamin B complex. Flavonoids especially polymethoxyflavones, flavanone glycosides, and limonoids are natural secondary metabolite compounds of citrus.

Fruits have a lot of biological effective compounds, that have the ability to attack radical free and work as anti-natural oxidative stress, such as phenolic compounds (phenolic acids, flavonoids, and tannins) make them play an important role in reducing the risk of many diseases like cancers, cardiovascular and neurological diseases.

Researchers say Samoan mamala tree bark tea could lead to HIV-AIDS cure

https://www.abc.net.au/news/2013-09-13/an-samoan-tree-bark-could-hold-key-to-hiv-cure/4955458

US scientists believe a synthetic version of a traditional Pacific medicine could hold the key to finding a cure for HIV-AIDS. In Samoa, traditional healers have long used the bark of the mamala

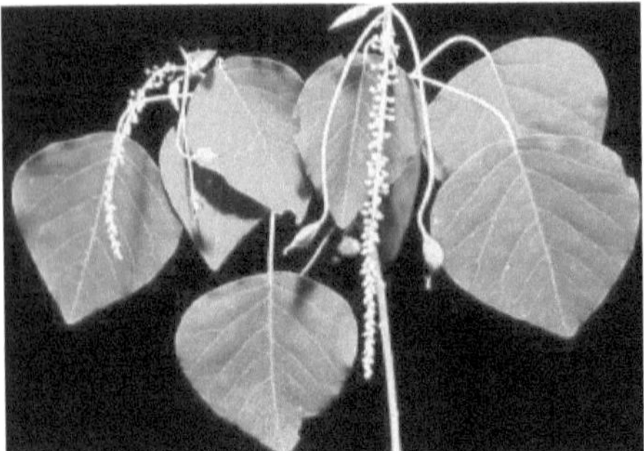

tree in tea to treat ailments such as hepatitis.

A recent meeting of the American Chemical Society was told the bark contains prostratin, which can be used to activate HIV viruses inside latent cells. Lead researcher, Professor Paul Wender, has told Radio Australia's Pacific Beat program that until now, the latent virus has been beyond the range of effective conventional treatments which target the active virus.

"What we hope to do is to get at the root of the disease, rather than snipping off leaves above ground, as is the case right now. It's very important to do, it stops progression of HIV-AIDS, but we need to get at the root," he said. "We know that current therapy... is able to keep the active virus under control - it suppresses the active virus to undetectable levels. But if one stops taking one's medications, that active virus is resupplied by the latent virus, so what we need to attack is the latent virus, the source of the active virus and that's what these compounds do."

Professor Wender's team has been working to create synthetic versions of prostratin which are 100 times as potent. The group is also developing synthetic versions of bryostatin, a substance that occurs in sea creatures called bryozoans. Professor Wender says the synthetic 'analogs' also allow compounds which are rare in nature to be used in large-scale treatment.

He says learning from nature could allow scientists to develop new treatments for a variety of conditions. "We can make things that are better than the natural product - that's not a position of arrogance, it simply means that nature's making these natural products and other materials for its own uses and its own ecosystem, not necessarily to treat AIDS or treat cancer or Alzheimer disease," he said. "But we could learn how nature is using these compounds, and then think about it - connect the dots - to the problems that we're trying to solve, and then modify them so they could do things that have never been done before. When we humans learned that it's the concavity of a bird's wing that allows the lift that allows for heavier than air flight, we didn't go off and synthesise a bird - so that's where we are at a molecular level with our research. We're studying what nature's doing with an eye toward using that solve unsolved problems."

6 reasons doctors say to avoid colon cleanses

https://www.cbc.ca/news/health/colonics-colon-cleanses-doc-tor-warning-hydrotherapy-1.4543340

'Trying to help along a system that's already perfected biologically is pointless': GI specialist says
Former customers of two colon cleansing services in Thunder Bay, Ont, are getting tested for Hepatitis B and C as well as HIV after complaints of poor hygiene practices at the businesses. The city's health unit is warning clients may have been exposed to improperly cleaned instruments by having the service.

Earlier this year, Gwyneth Paltrow's celebrity lifestyle website, Goop, recommended a do-it-yourself coffee enema to as a detox "supercharge." She also endorses colonics. But health experts say there is no scientific evidence to support colon cleaning treatments, which are popping up in Canadian cities.

What is it?
Colonics are also known as colon cleaning, colonic irrigation or colonic hydrotherapy. Colonic hygienists or colon therapists usu-

ally perform the procedure. People also perform it on themselves. It works like an enema but with much more fluid - up to 60 litres or 16 gallons. That's the equivalent of a gas tank in a Honda Civic. The patient usually lies on a table and water is slowly pumped into the rectum through a tube. Sometimes herbs or compounds are added. Fluids and waste are expelled.

Why do people do it?
Colonics are promoted as a way to clean out the colon of waste. "For things like weight loss, anti-aging and natural beauty there can be a lot of appeal," said Monica Black, who offers the service in Toronto and flushes her own colon monthly.

Dr. Ranit Mishori of Georgetown University School of Medicine in Washington, D.C. reviewed colon cleansing for a 2011 paper published in the Journal of Family Practice. People hear about it from a variety of celebrities like Paltrow, as well as internet and magazine marketing campaigns, she said. "I think they don't know that a) there are risks and b) that there's no evidence whatsoever behind all of these claims for feeling better, losing weight, battling depression, enhancing your immunity."
Mishori, a professor of family medicine, said in an interview with CBC News. "None of these things have been studied or have been proven to be correct in terms of the marketing."

What does the science say?
Stool is a waste product in and of itself and the colon does not build up toxins, said Dr. Constantine Soulellis, a gastroenterologist at the McGill University Health Centre in Montreal. "Trying to help along a system that's already perfected biologically is pointless," Soulellis said.

What are the risks?
In Mishori's review, complications ranged from: An imbalance of minerals and electrolytes such as salts after absorbing so much water. Electrolyte disturbances can lead to heart failure and kidney

damage. Interference with bacteria that are supposed to line the colon. Infection. Slight tears in the intestines to full perforations and even death. Soulellis has treated serious complications. "I did see a patient once with a colonic perforation and wound up with an ostomy," or a waste bag, he said. "The colon had to be diverted away from the rectal and anal area because of the damage that was done."

Other side effects include: Cramping, Bloating, Nausea, Vomiting, Diarrhea, Dizziness, Dehydration, Pancreatitis. There have been warnings about infection risk, such as the one issued by Thunder Bay's public health unit in the most recent case.

Who polices it?
Health Canada said it regulates the sale, advertising and importation for sale of licensed medical devices, including 10 colonic irrigators that are authorized for use before surgery. The clinics, however, are not always checked. Health Canada said it does not inspect clinics that perform colonic hydrotherapy. Most Canadian cities also don't. "There's no standard for cleanliness, there's no standard for sterilization," Soulellis said. "It's very much an issue of buyer beware."

Now this may not be accurate information given here bit I did share some light on the cure for HIV.

Can HIV go away on it's own?
After your immune system loses the battle with HIV, the flu like symptoms will go away. Doctors may call this the asymptomatic or clinical latent period. If you are taking medication and have healthy habits, your HIV infection may not progress any further.

How long can the virus stay undetected?
After contracting the virus, it takes up to 4-10 weeks to detect it in the blood. Sometimes, it takes longer to get detected through blood tests even up to six months.

What is the life expectancy of an HIV person?

This is different for each individual living with HIV.

As we all know some people can die within months of diagnosis, just the idea of having it can stress you out mentally and kill you physically but some people can live a fairly healthy, long life with regular anti-retro viral therapy.

What is a carrier of HIV/AIDS?

These words have no medical term or affiliation with being HIV negative or positive in any way or form, this is just one of the most popular words that is used among us from many years ago until present.

This is why we need to educate ourselves in this area and stop being blind to the facts where HIV/AIDS is concerned.

This however may be a much less fabricated medical term used for being HIV positive, meaning that the person is a carrier of HIV and gives it to other people.

What is a carrier? A person or thing that carries, hold or conveys something, transport to a place from one point to the next.
1. To carry - He supports his wife in carrying of baggage
2. To bring - She brought her husband back from the clinic
3. To take - She lay hold of his hands
4. To fetch - He carried a bucket of water for his wife
5. To bear - He bore the weight of his wife
6. To move- While he was having sex with his wife they both changed positions
7. Shift - He moved the chairs for his wife
8. Transfer - They both slept comfortable after moving to their new home
9. The goods can be sent by carrier
10. Letters can be sent by carrier

Do HIV carriers test negative? (HIV CARRIERS) (HIV BASICS)

https://www.thebody.com/article/hiv-carrirers-test-nega-tive-hiv-carriers-hiv-basics

Question

DO HIV carriers test negative?

(I did an HIV 1&2 test which came back negative but someone told me that I could still be a carrier. The test was done six (6) months after my last possible exposure.

Answer

Hello, There is no such thing as an "HIV carrier." See below.

Dr. Bob, is there such thing as HIV- carriers? Mar 13, 2007

Hello Doc, I have tested negative for HIV out to six months and believe I am negative per the recommendations of this site and my own doctor. However, yesterday I had a discussion with some co-workers that really freaked me out. I consider myself pretty educated on HIV but they sounded so convincing in their argument that I had to double check with you.

They stated that some people can test negative for HIV but have it dormant in their system and become carriers of the decease. Is this accurate? From everything that I have read you have to be HIV positive to transmit and have not read about dormant stages beyond 3-6 months. Please help me out doc, this sent my fears soaring again. I thought I had put all this HIV stuff behind me but they just pulled me back in.

Response from Dr. Frascino.

Hello, No, there is no such thin as a dormant HIV carrier. Likewise, there is no such thing as a vampire, the tooth fairy, the Easter Bunny or a compassionate conservative, no matter what your whacko co-worker may spout off about or what you may hear on Fox News!

Untreated HIV carriers transmit resistant viruses

https://www.sciencedaily.com/releases/2013/11/131118080920.htm

Human-Immunodeficiency Viruses that resist AIDS medicines are primarily transmitted by people who are not actually undergoing treatment. In order to prevent a spread of the resistant viruses increased efforts in prevention and early diagnosis of new infections are needed, as concluded by the Swiss HIV Cohort Study that is supported by the Swiss National Science Foundation (SNSF).

Around one in every ten newly infected HIV carriers in Switzerland has viruses that are resistant to at least one of the three classes of drugs used to treat AIDS. Contrary to previously held assumptions, resistant viruses are primarily transmitted by people who are not yet receiving treatment, according to the reports in "Clinical Infectious Diseases" from the researchers headed by Roger Kouyos and Huldrych Günthard at Zurich University Hospital.

Reconstruction of transmission chains: In their molecular epidemiological analysis of 1674 male carriers of HIV who had sex with other men, the researchers demonstrated resistant viruses in 140 patients. The research group reconstructed the transmission chains of these viruses on the basis of the patients' estimated infection dates and the degree of genetic relatedness of their blood-borne viruses. Most of the transmission chains commence in HIV carriers who were not yet undergoing treatment at the time at which the resistant viruses were transmitted.

"We were astonished to note that the resistant viruses are primarily brought into circulation by untreated people," said Günthard. "Previously we had assumed that the resistant viruses came from patients for whom treatment had failed as resistances were produced while treatment was ongoing."

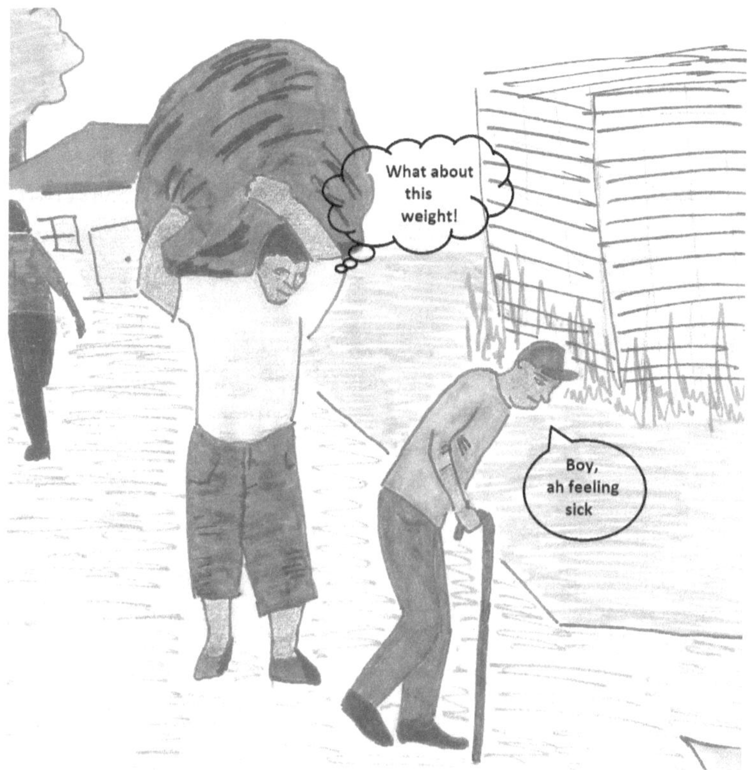

Early diagnosis is vital

The principal role of untreated HIV carriers in the transmission of resistant viruses means that combating these resistant strains is not solely reliant on optimised treatment, but also on preventing transmission by people who are not undergoing treatment. Prevention and early detection of newly infected persons are particularly vital in this respect. "In contrast to other tests, such as that for hepatitis, the HIV test requires that permission is obtained from the patient," explained Günthard. Since many doctors are reluctant to discuss their patients' sexuality with them openly, many infections are not discovered until much later than they could and should have been. While progress in medicine has robbed AIDS of its deadly effect, Günthard went on to stress, "there is still a great deal to be done."

The Swiss HIV Cohort Study
The aim of the study, which started in 1988, is to better understand HIV infection and AIDS, and improve the treatment of patients. All of Switzerland's specialist HIV clinics (Basel, Berne, Geneva, Lausanne, Lugano, St. Gallen and Zurich) collect data on treatment and the progress of the disease. Currently over 8,800 people are taking part in the Swiss HIV Cohort Study, of whom almost one third are women.

Record three in five HIV-carriers now have access to drugs: UN

https://medicalxpress.com/news/2018-07-hiv-carriers-access-drugs.html

Almost three in five people infected with HIV, or 21.7 million globally, took antiretroviral therapy in 2017—a new record for anti-AIDS drug access, the UN's HIV/AIDS agency said Wednesday. (July 2018)

There were 36.9 million people living with the immune system-attacking virus in 2017, of whom 15.2 million were not getting the drugs they need—the lowest number since the epidemic exploded, UNAIDS reported. Hailing progress in curbing new infections and deaths, the agency nevertheless lamented the mounting human toll: almost 80 million infections and 35.4 million lives lost since the first cases became known in the early 1980s.

Progress made to date risks being halted, even reversed, if funding and world attention is allowed to dwindle, the agency warned. "We are short $7 billion (six billion euros) per year to maintain our results and to achieve our objectives for 2020," UNAIDS executive director Michel Sidibe told AFP. "Without these resources, there is a big risk of the epidemic rebounding, of an increase in mortality due to AIDS," he said.

In 2017, about $20.6 billion was available for AIDS programmes in low- and middle-income countries which funded about 56 percent from their own budgets, said the report. Under Donald Trump, the US administration - a major funder of AIDS programmes historically, has threatened to cut spending. The UN goal is for 90 percent of all HIV-positive people to know their status by 2020. Of these, at least 90 percent must receive ART, and the HIV virus be suppressed in 90 percent of those.

Infections decline

Assessing progress towards the target, UNAIDS said 1.8 million people became newly infected with HIV in 2017. This was down from about 1.9 million the year before, and 3.4 million at the peak of the epidemic in 1996. Deaths declined from 990,000 to 940,000 year-on-year, compared to 1.9 million in 2005 and 1.4 million in 2010. The number of people on antiretroviral therapy (ART) grew from 19.4 million in 2016 to 21.7 million last year—up from a mere 611,000 in the year 2000 and 2.1 million in 2005, said the report released in the run-up to the International AIDS Conference in Amsterdam next week. This helped boost the number of people living with the virus from 36.3 million in 2016 to 36.9 million last year.

Despite more than three decades of research, there is no cure or vaccine and HIV-positive people have to take lifelong treatment that can be expensive and have nasty side-effects. ART inhibits the virus and can limit its spread between people—mainly through sex—but does not kill it.

'We haven't won yet,' UNAIDS reported large variation between world regions in the battle against the killer virus.

In the Middle East and north Africa, for example, less than a third of people with HIV have access to ARV, only 36 percent of those in eastern Europe and central Asia, and 40 percent in west and central Africa. For west and central Europe and North America, the number is 78 percent, with about 1.7 million out of 2.2 million infected people on ARV, said UNAIDS. In east and southern Africa—home to 53 percent of people living with HIV in the world—deaths declined by 42 percent from 2010 to 2017, thanks largely to the widespread rollout of treatment.

However, "there has been no reduction in AIDS-related mortality in eastern Europe and central Asia since 2010, and deaths from AIDS-related illness increased by 11 percent in the Middle East and North Africa," cautioned the report. "Some countries continue to concern us, such as Nigeria which accounts for about half of all new infections in west Africa," said Sidibe.

In Russia, he added, the epidemic "is becoming widespread. While it was concentrated among people who inject drugs, it is affecting the general population more and more."

Sidibe blamed punitive laws, which instead of offering drug users access to clean, uninfected needles, force them underground "hiding and infecting their partners."

He also highlighted the particular vulnerability of children and teenagers. About 180,000 minors were newly infected with HIV in 2017, and about 110,000 died of AIDS, yet more than 50 percent of under-15s had no access to treatment. "This is unacceptable," said Sidibe, who warned of creeping apathy and "complacency" in the fight against AIDS.

"We can win, but we haven't won yet," he said of the global battle.

Using Condoms for the right Reason
[https://www.webmd.com/]

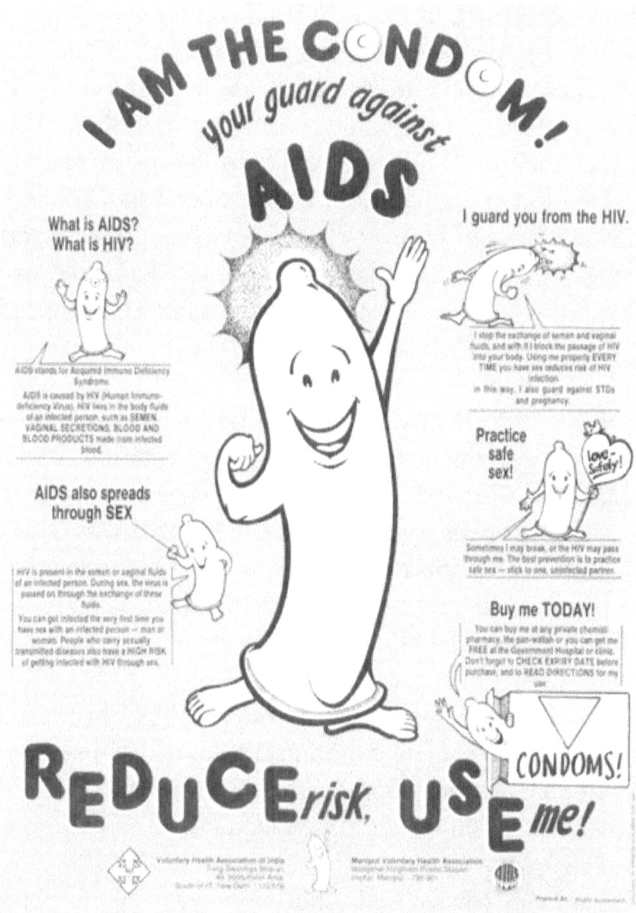

Condoms can protect you against sexually transmitted infections and can be used to prevent pregnancy. A male condom is placed over a man's erect penis before sex. Condoms are also called "rubber, sheaths, or skins." They are made of latex (rubber) polyurethane or sheep intestine.

Using condoms is not always 100% safe, many persons who promote condoms as a way of safe sex can not guarantee unwanted pregnancy and the prevention of sexually transmitted diseases. I write from experience, my cousin used condoms each and every time he had sex, his backyard was full of them. When I looked closely at these rubbers, every one of them were burst. When I asked him if he was an animal, he replied no man them thing dry rotting. Do you know how many children my cousin ended with? Ten children that is ten condom babies from using rubbers. Just name the condoms, he try every brand you could think of and each baby that was born is a mistake. So you see all them children was a mistake for him, all because of the condoms bursting while having sex.

Condoms are 98% effective in preventing pregnancy if used correctly. 86% on average includes pregnancies resulting from errors in condoms use. Condom breakage or slippage can occur around 2%, this rarely happens when condoms are properly used, fit is important. If it is too tight it may burst, when it is too loose then it will slip off. Not forgetting the female condom, you and I know very well it's not popular as much as male condoms in this country.

The male condom has a user failure rate of 18%. This means that among all couples that use condoms 18 out of 100 become pregnant in one year. Among couples who use condoms perfectly for 1 year, only 2 out of 100 will become pregnant.

"In Trinidad and Tobago and other parts of the world people fall in love, some at first sight others infatuation, in general couples use condoms for a week or less after hooking up and then they bang, bang. "Yes baby yes," - They are going skin on skin like dogs or rabbits.
- Some people make lame excuses for not using condoms, like:
"Baby look how long you know me, you feel I have AIDS, I clean."
"Honey you know I like it raw, it is sweeter that way."

"This thing does make meh uncomfortable, ah does like it when you cum on meh."

"Babes when you use a condom on meh, ah doh get de sensation ah doh feel nottin."

- Some women engage in unprotected sex for other reason like trapping a man with a baby.
- When you have a little to much alcohol, you are too drunk to wear condoms.
- Some men have too much anxiety when peeling off a condom, it's too much hustle while trying to put it on and the excitement make them have an erection, having to start all over again.
- When a woman or man ask the question: don't you love me? Yes is the reply and then it goes well "if" you love me we don't have to use that condom. They would say that because is only one thing they want.

Accidents do happen in bed but having unprotected sex is different, then you get pregnant, which you didn't plan for. The next step is to blame the partner, is your fault all this would not have happened if you did use a condom. In this situation both parties lay blame on each other.

With my cousin, however I really can't say why and how those condoms broke or burst with him while having sex with his wife. Male condoms are one of the best forms of birth-control out there because they are cheap, you can buy them anywhere, they prevent pregnancy and they also prevent the spread of sexually transmitted diseases but they only work if they don't break."**"**
There are six reasons why condoms might rip:
1. The condom is past its prime - condom wrappers have an expiration date on them, so be sure to take note.

2. Storage issues - Heat damages latex condoms, so they shouldn't be kept in hot places such as glove compartments or wallets. Keep

them in your chest of drawers or even under pillows which make it much easier to put your hands on.

3. Lack of lubrication - If there is friction while having sex, especially anal sex, not only will it cause pain and irritation to your privates, but the condom can also break. So be sure to use lubricated condoms or use extra lube if you need to.

4. You're using the wrong lubricant. If you're using latex condoms, oil-based lubricants can weaken the rubber and cause a tear, so use only water-based lubes.

5. The condom doesn't fit. If the condom is too small or too large, it can rip during rough sex, so experiment with different-sized condoms to get a snug fit - not too tight and not too loose.

6. The woman is tight. Some women vaginal muscles are naturally tight, so to help prevent condom breakage, lubrication (and a lot of it) is a must.

"This is what I have seen happening in our nation's schools. Condom (aka rubbers) distribution has been going on for years where private institutions like churches and government ministries are going around in different locations to hand out rubbers to male and female students. This is nothing new today.

Their belief is that in handing out the condoms to these students, that it will give them a sense of confidence and a way of protection to have a thing they call safe sex. Whatever the situation may be, this approach could be inappropriate for me as it is a way of encouraging and engaging them to go have fun now, with permission to have lots of intercourse. This is a good way for them to experiment and gain experience.

Which is more important? A good academic foundation towards

a better education first, for a better future generation or condoms, rubbers, sex education for the next generation? Which may produce a negative stigma on our school system especially towards new born babies and HIV infections.

Apart from all these condoms or no condoms, sex education or normal education does not divert students from engaging in unprotected sexual intercourse.

1. First of all are these students being taught by a tutor or a medical practitioner?

2. Some of these students don't even have an idea what is the proper use of a condom and type.

3. Condom distribution without proper advice to those students may send the wrong signal to both male and female students.

Then we have the parents who have a big part to play in this situation. Teachers and governments are not to blame for this, it starts at home. Yes, where they live and what we do as parents in front of our children. For example single mothers who are poor, and can't afford books, uniform, shoes, book bags etc. They cannot provide money for their daughter to go back and forth to school, now this will bring a tremendous stress and frustration between mother and daughter.

In cases mammy will now invite a little boy-friend at night to sleep over knowing her daughter's room is next to hers. What you think will happen? She's going to hear everything that mammy is doing in the room. This girl now is saying, if mammy could have man, I could have a man too.

I need you to see the picture here, her mother has a man for the purpose of financial gains, a way to provide for her daughter but it is sending the wrong signal to this girl. This was a reference of what is taking place in our country.

In this true story I tell of how I got to know my children's mother. There were three sisters living together with their mother, no father because there was a separation, you will know later on. What I remember is that these three girls would travel to come down the road almost every day when I had the shop. One of them would come into my shop regularly and we would talk. Now, she was the eldest of the three, this went on for about a year. She was eighteen going on nineteen, while speaking to these three young girls the kind of things that I was hearing, it was unbelievable.

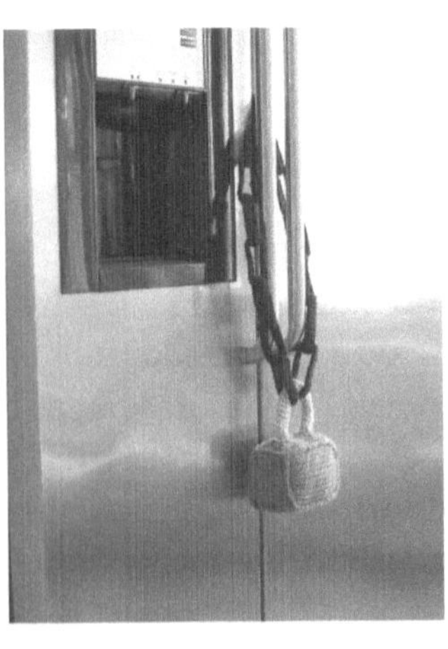

These were the exact words: "Mummy does put chain around the handle of the refrigerator with a padlock and we does not have anything to eat. We does go on the mango tree to pick mango and eat, sometimes on the guava tree."

I used to buy pizza or give them money to get things in order for them to cook food. This went on for a good while until I find it was time to talk to their mother about the nonsense she was doing and it was girls not boys. After meeting their mother, telling her about the situation with the girls you know she told me that they lying on her, that they not telling the truth.

Okay, I left it at that for a while.

I waited until she left the country, you know the girls decided to carry me home to see for myself. Upon reaching at their home the first place they took me was in the kitchen. To my surprise there

160

was a chain and a padlock around the refrigerator and the cupboards in the kitchen, every one was empty.

I decided it was time to ask about their father and why he was separated from them.
"Mummy used to be in the bedroom with man when daddy gone
to work and we hearing mummy screaming and the door banging," these were their exact words.

"Are you sure and how do you know?" I asked.

They replied that there was a hole in the door where they would
peep and see everything. Then there was another occasion with the
guava tree shaking and they were thinking it was the breeze only
to see their mother holding on to the tree having sex with a man.

These girls continue to say the kinds of things they would hear going on with their mother was shameful and embarrassing. Which
is why their father had to leave and go. This is how my children's
mother and I met, I was in my late twenties and was feeling sorry
for the girls, after some time we developed a relationship and I
took her away.

For me this was a wicked act for a mother to do to her three girls.
She could afford to give them food and money because this lady
had money, she did good business.

Where on the other-hand some poor single mothers can't afford to
give their daughters anything. With situations like these, children
at an early age would have dropped out of school, others may have
also gotten pregnant very early. Hence the reason why these young
girl go home with a new $700 sneakers or earrings and when their
mother asked them; "Girl whey yuh get that from? Or Where did
you get the money to buy that? They reply, "but mammy is uncle
John wha give meh that." Now many mothers will never call uncle

John to really find out if he purchased those items and that will remain dead for a long time. What will happen after when John realize that mammy eh jumbie-in[24] him, it is obvious they both will take it to the next level by exchanging phone numbers and so on.

"When yuh leaving home put some extra clothes and underwear in yuh school bag."

Eventually she will start coming home late from the usual time school would over. Upon reaching home a little late:

"Girl why you coming home this hour?"

"Oh gosh mammy ah was taking extra lessons because I have exams coming up so ah need this extra lesson. Ah was supposed to let you know, ah forgot."

A couple of months down the road meh girl stop seeing she period or monthly's (menstrual cycle), being in mammy house you could hide but not for long, it have a thing called morning sickness, nausea and vomiting. So mammy must know and then what? Here is the thing:

"Girl who is de man?"

"...But mammy," "Girl doh tell meh nottin yuh hear, what yuh go tell meh eh what?"
"...But mammy you ain't listening,"

"Let meh hear you."
"Mammy is John, is John who do meh dat."

"... But I thought was yuh uncle, look nah!"

"No mammy, ah was afraid yuh would ah beat meh."

"So what then girl?"

"Mammy ah doh know."

"Girl you see what problems alyuh does bring eh, ah done have enough on meh already. What about school eh? You not studying home here, if you have to band up your belly you going," Says her mother.

*****

There is this school in my area where children will come to school with a change of clothes in their bags for the purpose of liming. Some of these activities do take place during school hours or after, these students will go under bridges or in the hills at the back of the school where there are nearby bushes to have sex. Not only in this school but throughout the country have similar issues, within a few months some schools will have doctors to have these students take pregnancy tests and the number of girls that was found pregnant is not good at all.

In those days my mother and father used to tell us when we ask question about how we were born: "Boy you drop from a breadfruit tree or you fall from a flying plane, boy you fall from the sky," and all that nonsense.

In the old days we have to learn on our own. Where in today's world the younger generation are born into having ideas before hand.

Parents must teach their children about sex, the good, the bad and the ugly part and consequences. **"**

References

Country Fact Sheets

Trinidad and Tobago 2017
HIV and AIDS Estimates

Adults and children living with HIV	11 000 [9600 - 12 000]
Adults aged 15 and over living with HIV	11 000 [9500 - 12 000]
Women aged 15 and over living with HIV	3900 [3500 - 4300]
Men aged 15 and over living with HIV	6800 [5800 - 7600]
Children aged 0 to 14 living with HIV	<200 [<200 - <200]

UNAIDS has estimated that as of 2017 there are approximately 11,000 persons living with HIV in Trinidad and Tobago. It further estimates that since the start of the epidemic in 1983 to present there have been fever than 23,000 persons diagnosed with HIV (data to 2016).

In our country the statistics for 2015 was 10,800 reported. This was an estimate of all persons - including adult and children alive at the year-end with an HIV infection. However, in 2016 that figure increased to 11,000 (9800-12000) and in 2017 remained the same. They estimate that there is almost one person in every family in Trinidad and Tobago living with HIV.

A study in Denmark (2005) estimated that the survival rate is more than thirty-five years for a young person diagnosed with HIV and another study in Canada (2003) has shown that life expectancy at the age of twenty was an additional 58.3 years. Studies here and the world over has shown that persons can live with HIV for 20 - 70 years. In 2012, the HIV prevalence rate was 1.5% indicating that Trinidad and Tobago is categorized as having a generalized epidemic due to our ratio to population of 1.3 million and infected persons of 22,085 at the time. I really don't know how accurate this information is, but people like Mr. Fabulous with treatment had HIV for ten years, he was twenty-eight when he contracted it. He only lived to be thirty-eight but I can't say if he was ever off the medication or if he took it as he should. Again, I don't know how accurate the information is for Trinidad because I have seen many people who lived for shorter periods than the figure mentioned here.

You can compare the statistics for yourself and see that it wasn't always possible over the years.

God never intended for us to have or come in contact with this virus, it is because of sin. In the book of Genesis 2:18 God said : "It is not good for a man to be alone. I will make a helper that is suitable for him."

God made all things, he made us to choose right from wrong, life or death. So if we choose the path of sin which is not of God, these are the consequences for sin. Having more than one woman, man with man. God destroyed a city for these reasons. Sodom and Gomorrah (Genesis (18 -20 v 22:33).

Romans 1:24-29 - "and likewise also the men, leaving the natural use of woman, burned in their lust on towards another, men with men working that which is unseemly and receiving in themselves that recompense of their error which was meet and even as they did not like to retain God in their knowledge."

God give them over to a reprobate mind, to do those things which are not convenient. Being filled with all unrighteousness, fornication, wickedness, covetousness, maliciousness, full of envy, murder, debate, deceit, malignity, whisperers.

CLOSING

This book is dedicated in memory of all those wonderful people who passed on but are not forgotten. Like anyone else they took a chance risking their lives by putting trust in persons by having sex with them. Hence the reason why HIV/AIDS was contacted from one person to the other, leaving them with no choice but to take medical treatment in order to survive for a while until their immune system gave way. This is really a part of life that we must face.

As I remember and I give you my closing statement that having an estimate of persons or places, all who were and is involved with the deadly disease are countless and horrifying. For what my eyes had seen so many people that were known to me who lived with HIV over a period of time are dead and some are alive today still fighting the battle with treatment just to stay alive.

Again, I am hoping and praying that some people will be able to read and understand from the mistake of others, my question from years ago to present is: Is this an epidemic waiting to get out of control? Or is it already out of control? Only God knows for there are many people in our society today who are walking around with HIV/AIDS and are afraid to get tested knowing what the results may be.

There are those who are going to churches and getting married without taking this test, hoping and putting their trust in God, even though we are true in heart to do the right thing, still go get tested. In that way people lives will be saved and safe. Don't take people life with yours as a revenge on innocent ones.

Now, all these situations were as a result of unfaithfulness, covetousness, cheating with other people, horning one another husband or wife, this is just an excited experiment with great price to pay on your life.

People, these times are not for games playing and fooling around. All is infatuation in our head trying to get out that satisfaction of a never-ending ego. For me you either stay single or have a committed partner that you are sure about which may lead to marriage.

Please take precaution, no one can take responsibility for you and your foolish actions. Stop blaming others for what has already been done, live right, be faithful to your man or woman, don't wait until you get HIV to say like others: "If ah did know."

Most importantly please stop the stigma against people who are living with HIV/AIDS, put yourself in their position and you will want to be treated likewise, after all they are as human just like the rest of us. Remember they did not ask for it and this can happen to anyone of us. Some took chances and were fortunate, others were not. We are not perfect but for God's sake stop wondering and go get tested. This is the only way you will know, forget others and what they may say and just think of your health.

Doctors do try their very best to treat you. HIV/AIDS is a killer for men, women, boys and girls. This deadly disease has no limits of age or gender just like drugs, say no. Say no to oral sex in the office areas, say no to spontaneous sex in public places, say no to sex out of marriage. Most of all say no to sex without condoms.

Remember prevention is much better than cure.

GIVE
AIDS A

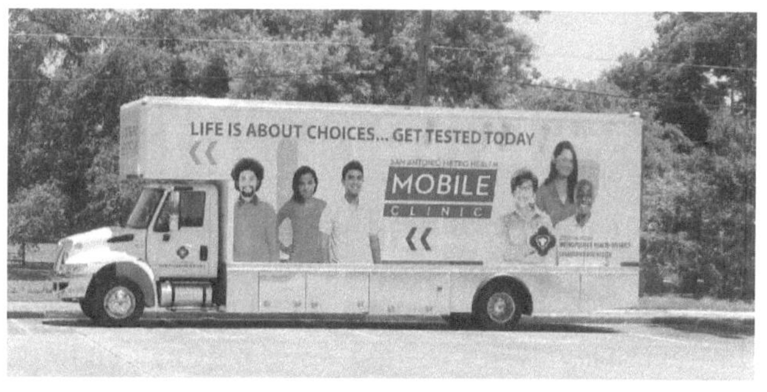

About the Author

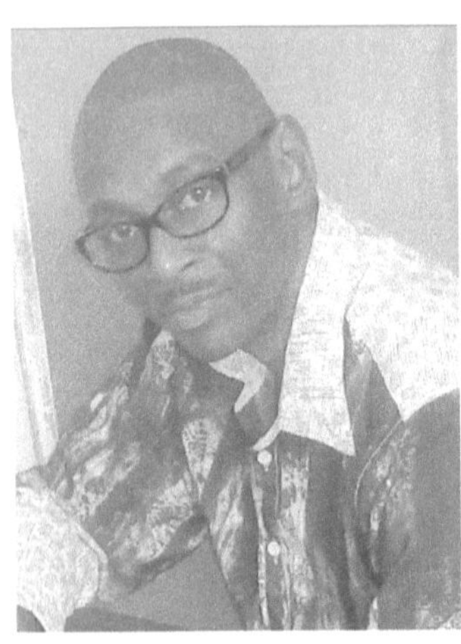

Karcian Suragh is a first-time author. His book HIV/AIDS Why me? Is ah chance ah go take, is a compilation of true stories depicting the lives of persons before they contracted the HIV virus.

Suragh was born in Trinidad and Tobago in 1966 and attended San Juan Boys RC, then San Juan Private Secondary school. Born to Grenadian and Vincentian parents he had many hobbies such as electronics, cooking, listening to music of any genre, meeting people from all cultures, hiking, camping out, going to the beach, window shopping and of course writing. At the end of secondary school, Suragh tried out for the Trinidad and Tobago Fire Service at the same time of his final exams, both areas suffered and he switched to an Electronics Technician Technologies course. He remembers his hatred for mathematics in school because of a teacher who would beat anyone who didn't know the answer but he had to face math once again as he excelled at electronics and became an entrepreneur. Electronics gain was indeed the writing world's loss as Suragh excelled as a technician and pushed writing aside as a mere hobby for over fifteen years. He also wanted to be a geologist in his early twenties because of his love for nature and God's handiwork. His passion however was always writing, since putting pen to paper at night may be his favourite past time. He says it's a beautiful thing to have a story to tell. He went on to write skits for plays, short stories and now is a published author.

Today as a single father to two boys he would return to this manuscript determined to publish it for it's relevance to the world today, especially after seeing people caught up within triangle relationships, falling in love, not knowing theirs or their partners HIV status or intentions, sometimes getting infected by persons who were HIV positive.

In times past, friends would gather and somehow the conversation always moved to the topic of HIV/AIDS. Everyone knew of someone who had the disease and would discuss the matter, when it was his turn he would speak about Mr. Fabulous and everyone would ask: Who is he? What country did this happen? When they realize it all happened in Trinidad and Tobago they remained surprised. Suragh realized that people wanted to know and learn more about HIV/AIDS prevention, awareness, the proper uses of condoms and what safe sex really was. Knowing that young people were sexually active gave him the drive to publish his book and stop just talking about doing it. He wants people to be educated on HIV/AIDS in a different manner, not just once a year but daily, weekly, and monthly because people have sex in the same instances which allows this deadly disease to spread faster than we think which is why he thinks HIV/AIDS prevention should be taught in all schools. He notes that compiling HIV/AIDS risk and sexual behaviour in both men and women over the last two decades was an inspiration to write. He believes that there is a hidden ability in each one of us and when you discover it you should use it wisely.

This book is a keepsake for all who purchase it.

Other Books in the Series

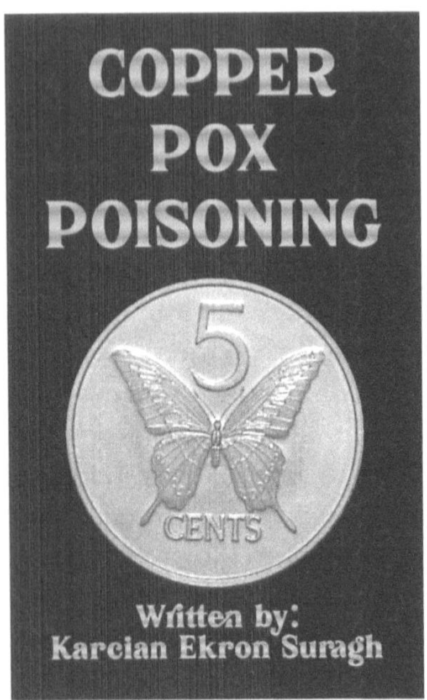

When I first came across this unusual subject it was more than four decades ago, during my early teens. My next-door neighbor was terminally ill with copper pox poisoning. Strange enough as a present witness then to Mr. Ben's pain and suffering, I remembered he offered the doctor the sum of ten thousand dollars in cash or any amount to get him better. The doctor refused, he told Ben he was unable and couldn't

help him.

I never forgot that day and spent many years investigating this strange illness. It felt more like superstition at times but weird as this may sound, copper pox poisoning is a very real disease unknown to the world and it has no cure whatsoever.

COMING SOON
INJUSTICES